# Pediatric Neurology

## What Do I Do Now?

SERIES CO-EDITORS-IN-CHIEF

Lawrence C. Newman, MD
Director of the Headache Institute
Department of Neurology
St. Luke's-Roosevelt Hospital Center
New York, New York

Morris Levin, MD
University of California
San Francisco

OTHER VOLUMES IN THE SERIES
Headache and Facial Pain
Peripheral Nerve and Muscle Disease
Pediatric Neurology
Stroke
Epilepsy
Neuro-ophthalmology
Neuroimmunology
Pain
Neuroinfections
Emergency Neurology
Cerebrovascular Disease
Movement Disorders
Neurogenetics
Neurotology

# Pediatric Neurology

## SECOND EDITION

Gregory L. Holmes, MD
Professor and Chair of Neurological Sciences
University of Vermont
Burlington, Vermont

Peter M. Bingham, MD
Professor of Neurological Sciences and Pediatrics
University of Vermont
Burlington, Vermont

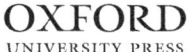

**OXFORD**
UNIVERSITY PRESS

Oxford University Press is a department of the University of Oxford. It furthers
the University's objective of excellence in research, scholarship, and education
by publishing worldwide. Oxford is a registered trade mark of Oxford University
Press in the UK and certain other countries.

Published in the United States of America by Oxford University Press
198 Madison Avenue, New York, NY 10016, United States of America.

© Oxford University Press 2016

First Edition published in 2010
Second Edition published in 2016

All rights reserved. No part of this publication may be reproduced, stored in
a retrieval system, or transmitted, in any form or by any means, without the
prior permission in writing of Oxford University Press, or as expressly permitted
by law, by license, or under terms agreed with the appropriate reproduction
rights organization. Inquiries concerning reproduction outside the scope of the
above should be sent to the Rights Department, Oxford University Press, at the
address above.

You must not circulate this work in any other form
and you must impose this same condition on any acquirer.

Library of Congress Cataloging-in-Publication Data
Names: Holmes, Gregory L., author. | Bingham, Peter M., author.
Title: Pediatric neurology / Gregory L. Holmes, Peter M. Bingham.
Other titles: What do I do now?
Description: Second edition. | Oxford ; New York : Oxford University Press, 2016. |
Series: What do I do now? | Includes bibliographical references and index.
Identifiers: LCCN 2015044626 | ISBN 9780190601508 (paperback : alk. paper) |
ISBN 9780190601522 (e-book) | ISBN 9780190601515 (e-book) | ISBN 9780190601539 (online)
Subjects: | MESH: Child—Case Reports. | Nervous System Diseases—Case Reports. |
Adolescent—Case Reports. | Infant—Case Reports.
Classification: LCC RJ486 | NLM WS 340 | DDC 618.92/8—dc23
LC record available at http://lccn.loc.gov/2015044626

9 8 7 6 5 4 3 2 1
Printed by Webcom, Canada

This material is not intended to be, and should not be considered, a substitute for medical or other
professional advice. Treatment for the conditions described in this material is highly dependent on
the individual circumstances. And, while this material is designed to offer accurate information
with respect to the subject matter covered and to be current as of the time it was written, research
and knowledge about medical and health issues is constantly evolving and dose schedules for
medications are being revised continually, with new side effects recognized and accounted for
regularly. Readers must therefore always check the product information and clinical procedures
with the most up-to-date published product information and data sheets provided by the
manufacturers and the most recent codes of conduct and safety regulation. The publisher and the
authors make no representations or warranties to readers, express or implied, as to the accuracy or
completeness of this material. Without limiting the foregoing, the publisher and the authors make
no representations or warranties as to the accuracy or efficacy of the drug dosages mentioned in the
material. The authors and the publisher do not accept, and expressly disclaim, any responsibility
for any liability, loss or risk that may be claimed or incurred as a consequence of the use and/or
application of any of the contents of this material.

## Acknowledgment

We are grateful to Mo Levin and Larry Newman for instigating the earlier edition of the *What Do I Do Now?—Pediatric Neurology* series. Craig Panner and Rebecca Suzan from Oxford University Press were very supportive in the planning and completion of this work. Most of all, we thank our patients and our colleagues at the University of Vermont Children's Hospital, who continue to teach us much about pediatric neurology.

*Gregory L. Holmes*
*Peter M. Bingham*
Burlington, Vermont

# Preface

Pediatric neurology is a challenging yet fascinating discipline that studies neurological diseases in a growing and maturing nervous system. The variety of clinical presentations, responses to therapy, and outcomes all reflect the highly plastic, impressionable nature of the developing human nervous system. Considering the evolving nature of clinical work and practice standards in this field, it is timely and appropriate for the editors to provide an updated edition of *What Do I Do Now?* Pediatric Neurology.

The 31 cases that make up this book come from our experience as pediatric neurologists over the past 30 years. Pediatric neurology has developed into a broad specialty, incorporating disciplines ranging from neuromuscular disease to neurogenetics to neurometabolic disorders. The cases presented here represent a mere snapshot of some common and some less common disorders encountered by pediatric neurologists. This book is by no means a comprehensive review of any of the topics; rather, we compare this book to wine tasting, where one can sample wine in small aliquots; the interested reader gets a brief taste of a variety of pediatric cases. The scenarios are designed to entice the reader to consider what he or she would do next. While we have included lists of differential diagnoses for many of the cases, most astute clinicians can reduce the differential diagnosis to a few possibilities after taking a history and performing an examination. We have therefore purposely tried to eliminate rare and unlikely conditions from the differential diagnoses.

This book is targeted toward pediatricians, family practitioners, adult neurologists, medical students, and nurse practitioners. Most of the cases presented here could be managed by interested healthcare professionals without formal pediatric neurology training, as in many parts of the country pediatric neurologists aren't readily available for consultation. Each case is short, encompassing salient features of the diagnosis. The cases are not meant to be tricky or misleading.

We hope this book will convey our own excitement as we work on a daily basis with children with neurological disorders. Ideally this book will motivate readers to dig deeper into the literature to learn more about the disorders. If this book is successful in helping even a single child with a neurological disorder, the effort will have been worthwhile.

*Gregory L. Holmes, MD*
*Peter M. Bingham, MD*
Burlington, Vermont

# Contents

### SECTION I PAROXYSMAL DISORDERS

1. The Girl Who Wouldn't Answer  3
2. Ephemeral Weakness: Which Side Are You On?  9
3. Newborn with a Rhythmic Twitch  15
4. Muteness at Breakfast  21
5. Going Limp: A Case of Recurring Collapse  27
6. Autonomic Storms En Route  33
7. A Frightful Awakening  39
8. Beyond Colic: The Distant Infant  45
9. The Twitch That Came Before  53
10. Airway, Breathing, Circulation, and Anticonvulsants  61

### SECTION II CONGENITAL AND GENETIC DISORDERS

11. A Question of Family History  69
12. Of Cramped Limbs and a Rough Start  75
13. The Case of the Changing Gait  81
14. The Boy Who Couldn't Keep Up  87
15. Beyond Autism: A Genetic Resolution  93
16. Learning Difficulty: Diagnosis Beyond the Neurological Examination  97
17. A Sleepy Newborn  105
18. A Loss of Connection  113
19. The Weak Baby  119
20. Contents Under Pressure  125
21. Episodic Weakness: Seeing Through the Smoke  133

## SECTION III POTPOURRI: INFLAMMATORY, PAIN, NEUROPSYCHIATRIC, AND MOVEMENT DISORDERS

22 **A Panoply of Symptoms** 141

23 **The Girl with the Bizarre Gait** 147

24 **Heavy Legs and a Sore Back** 153

25 **A Sudden Loss of Balance** 159

26 **Darting Eyes** 165

27 **Walking on Tiptoes** 171

28 **The Boy Who Kept Rolling His Eyes** 177

29 **A Sudden Collapse** 183

30 **The Headache That Wouldn't Go Away** 189

31 **Headache: To Scan, or Not to Scan?** 195

**Index** 201

# SECTION I
# Paroxysmal Disorders

# 1 The Girl Who Wouldn't Answer

You are called by a pediatrician who is seeing a 7-year-old girl with staring episodes. According to the pediatrician, teachers have noted the child stares off into space frequently. During the episodes the girl does not respond to questions. The pediatrician suspects the child is daydreaming but calls you to see if he should obtain an EEG.

**What do you do now?**

## ABSENCE SEIZURES

When questioned about a child who is having staring episodes, the physician should consider daydreaming, attention-deficit/hyperactivity disorder (ADHD), a sleep disorder, or a seizure disorder. The correct diagnosis can usually be made by asking a few questions. The family or teacher should be asked:

- Is a motor arrest witnessed, or is the child more often "discovered" in the midst of staring?
- Can the episodes be terminated by questioning or touching the child?
- Are there any motor signs during the event?
- Does the child quickly return to baseline after the event?
- How long do the episodes last?

Absence seizures are generalized seizures, indicating bi-hemispheric initial involvement clinically and on EEG. Absence seizures have an abrupt onset and offset. There is typically a sudden cessation of activities with a blank, distant look to the face. As the seizure continues, there are often automatisms and mild clonic motor activity such as jerks of the arms and eye blinking. It is unusual for a child with typical absence seizures to simply stare without any other behavioral manifestations. An absence seizure typically lasts less than 30 seconds, usually less than 10 seconds.

Focal seizures with impairment of consciousness or awareness (formerly termed complex partial seizures) may begin with an aura and then progress to a period of unresponsiveness. As in absence seizures, focal seizures with impairment of consciousness or awareness are associated with automatisms such as lip smacking or gestures of the hands. Focal seizures with impairment of consciousness or awareness are longer than absence seizures, typically averaging 1 to 2 minutes, and are often followed by a period of confusion and tiredness.

Daydreaming usually occurs in a child who is bored. The child may stare but does not have the distinct change in facial expression seen in children with seizures. Motor activity does not occur during daydreaming and there is no post-staring confusion or tiredness. Usually, witnesses do not report an abrupt onset of behavioral staring events, and the child can be redirected with questions. Children with ADHD, while inattentive, typically do not have long periods of staring, unless they are overmedicated. As with daydreaming, ADHD is not associated with motor activity or post-staring impairment. Children with autism frequently have episodes of staring. While the EEG in autistic spectrum disorder is often abnormal, paroxysmal changes are more often compatible with focal seizures in this group.

It is important for any physician seeing a child with staring spells to have the child hyperventilate for 3 minutes. Even toddlers can sometimes be coaxed into hyperventilating with a pinwheel. A very high percentage of children with untreated absence seizures will have an absence seizure with hyperventilation. It is far less likely that hyperventilation will elicit a seizure in a child with focal seizures.

If the physician is concerned that the child has epilepsy, an EEG can be very useful. The EEG signature of a typical absence seizure is the sudden onset of 3-Hz generalized symmetrical spike or multiple spike-and-wave complexes (Fig. 1–1). The EEG should include hyperventilation, photic

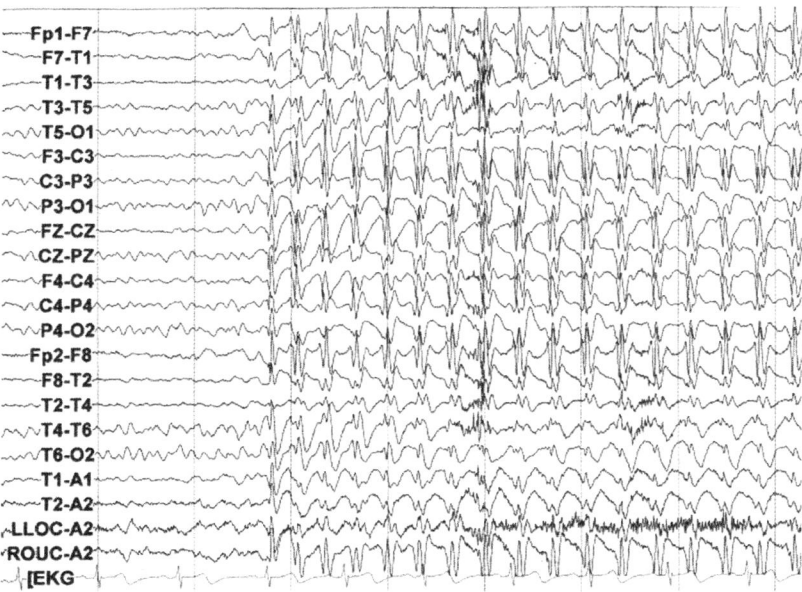

**FIGURE 1-1** Generalized spike-and-wave discharge in a 7-year-old with absence seizures.

stimulation, and sleep, any of which may increase the likelihood of seeing generalized spike-and-wave activity.

Children with focal seizures with impairment of consciousness or awareness are more likely to have temporal or frontal lobe spikes (Fig. 1–2). A normal EEG during wakefulness, sleep, hyperventilation, and photic stimulation would make the diagnosis of absence seizures quite unlikely. However, children with focal seizures can have normal EEGs. Table 1.1 provides a summary of key differentiating points between absence seizures, focal seizures with impairment of consciousness or awareness, daydreaming, and ADHD.

After making the diagnosis, appropriate therapy can be initiated. For absence seizures, treatment with ethosuximide, valproate, or lamotrigine should be considered. In the case of focal seizures the range of drugs that could be used is much broader.

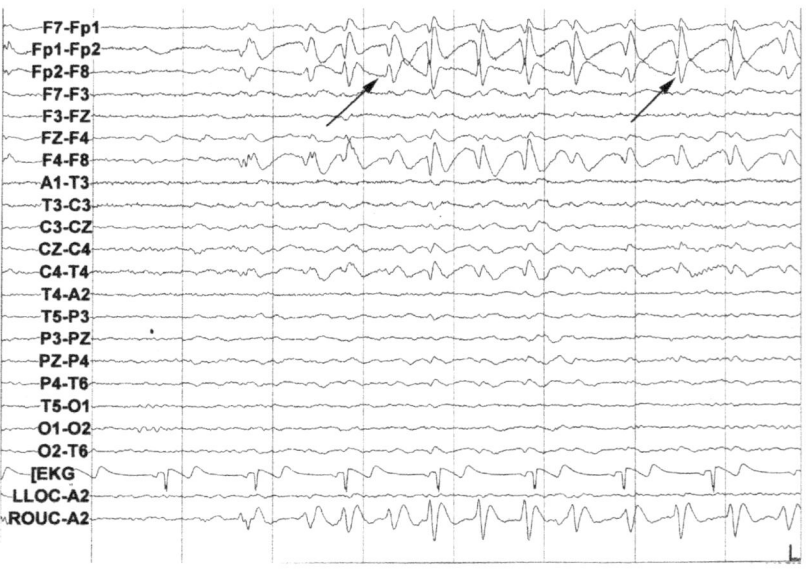

**FIGURE 1–2** Right frontal sharp waves (*arrows*) in a 9-year-old with focal seizures.

TABLE 1.1 **Differential Diagnosis of Staring Attacks**

|  | Absence Seizure | Focal Seizures with Impairment of Consciousness or Awareness | Daydreaming | ADHD |
|---|---|---|---|---|
| Aura | No | Frequently | No | No |
| Duration | <30 seconds | 1–2 minutes | Minutes | Seconds |
| Automatisms | Frequently | Frequently | No | No |
| Frequency | Multiple daily | Infrequent, unusual to have >2/day | Frequent, situation-dependent | Frequent |
| Post-staring impairment | No | Yes | No | No |
| EEG | Generalized spike-and-wave | Normal or focal discharges | Normal | Normal |

### KEY POINTS TO REMEMBER

- It is unusual for staring to be the only manifestation of an absence seizure.
- Must be differentiated from focal seizures with impairment of consciousness or awareness and non-epileptic events
- Seizures are short but occur frequently.
- Readily diagnosed with hyperventilation
- EEG shows generalized spike-and-wave activity in most cases.

Further Reading

Adams DJ, Lueders H. Hyperventilation and six-hour EEG recording in evaluation of absence seizures. *Neurology* 1981;31:1175–7.

Berg AT, Levy SR, Testa FM, Blumenfeld H. Long-term seizure remission in childhood absence epilepsy: might initial treatment matter? *Epilepsia* 2014;55:551–7.

Browne TR, Penry JK, Porter RJ, et al. Responsiveness before, during, and after spike-wave paroxysms. *Neurology* 1974;24:659–65.

Camfield C, Camfield P. Management guidelines for children with idiopathic generalized epilepsy. *Epilepsia* 2005;46(Suppl 9):112–6.

Camfield P, Camfield C. Epileptic syndromes in childhood: clinical features, outcomes, and treatment. *Epilepsia* 2002;43 (Suppl 3):27–32.

Glauser TA, Cnaan A, Shinnar S, et al. Ethosuximide, valproic acid, and lamotrigine in childhood absence epilepsy. *N Engl J Med* 2010;362:790–9.

Grosso S, Galimberti D, Vezzosi P, et al. Childhood absence epilepsy: evolution and prognostic factors. *Epilepsia* 2005;46:1796–801.

Holmes GL, McKeever M, Adamson M. Absence seizures in children: clinical and electroencephalographic features. *Ann Neurol* 1987;21:268–273.

Pavone P, Bianchini R, Trifiletti RR, et al. Neuropsychological assessment in children with absence epilepsy. *Neurology* 2001;56:1047–51.

Rosenow F, Wyllie E, Kotagal P, et al. Staring spells in children: descriptive features distinguishing epileptic and nonepileptic events. *J Pediatr* 1998;133:660–3.

Sato S, Dreifuss FE, Penry JK, et al. Long-term follow-up of absence seizures. *Neurology* 1983;33:1590–5.

# 2 Ephemeral Weakness: Which Side Are You On?

You are consulted by parents who believe their 7-year-old son has been incorrectly diagnosed with epilepsy. The parents tell you they became concerned about the child during the first year of life when he was felt to be more "floppy" than their two other children at a similar age. They also noted that the child was delayed in regards to sitting and walking and had bizarre, darting eye movements. During the second year the boy began having episodes where he would develop the sudden onset of right- or left-sided weakness. The weakness would last minutes to hours. The weakness would sometimes seem to alternate between the right and left side during the same attack. The boy was diagnosed with epilepsy by the neurologist. However, the parents said the neurologist was puzzled by the fact that EEGs during the attacks failed to show clear seizures.

The neurologist concluded that the seizures must be arising from a focus deep in the brain.

Over the years the parents described episodes of eye jerking and problems with balance. The child is now quite delayed and is receiving special educational services. He currently is taking clonazepam, valproate, and lamotrigine. The family feels these drugs, as with previous trials of other antiepileptic drugs in their son, have not reduced the number of attacks, although they believe that clonazepam has made the attacks less severe and shorter in duration.

You ask to examine the child, and note that he has a short attention span with poor eye contact. He speaks slowly and is dysarthric. He has nystagmus, which increases on lateral gaze bilaterally and has a rotatory component. He has diffuse hypertonia, hyperreflexia, and ataxia. During the examination he has an attack where his right arm drops to his side and he begins to bend to the right. When he starts crying you note that he has no clear facial weakness. The attack lasts about 10 minutes and resolves without any intervention.

### What do you do now?

## ALTERNATING HEMIPLEGIA OF CHILDHOOD

This child has alternating hemiplegia of childhood. It is not surprising that the neurologist made an incorrect diagnosis since this is a very rare condition that often mimics epilepsy. Indeed, some children may also have epilepsy as a distinct manifestation of the disorder, whose predominant features include episodic hypotonia, lateralized weakness, and episodic dystonia, usually superimposed on a global developmental delay. The EEG is often abnormal (variable slowing) but during the hemiplegia attacks there are no ictal discharges. Most, but not all, cases harbor a mutation in a gene that relates to function of a $Na^+/K^+$ ATPase channel, ATP1A3. Thus there is no uniformly reliable laboratory diagnostic test for alternating hemiplegia, and the diagnosis rests primarily on clinical criteria for this sporadically arising disorder. Spontaneous mutations of ATP1A3 can often be identified. ATP1A3 may also underlie other disorders, including rapid-onset dystonia/parkinsonism; episodic ataxia; and cerebellar ataxia, areflexia, pes cavus, optic atrophy, and sensorineural hearing loss (CAPOS) syndrome.

There are seven criteria for the diagnosis of alternating hemiplegia of childhood:

1. Onset before 18 months of age
2. Repeated episodes of hemiplegia involving the right or left side of the body
3. Episodes of bilateral hemiplegia or quadriplegia
4. Other paroxysmal disturbances, including tonic/dystonic attacks, nystagmus, strabismus, dyspnea, and other autonomic phenomena during hemiplegic attacks or in isolation
5. Immediate disappearance of all symptoms on going to sleep, with recurrence 10 to 20 minutes after awakening in long-lasting attacks
6. Evidence of developmental delay, learning disability, neurological abnormalities, choreoathetosis, dystonia, or ataxia
7. Not attributed to another disorder

As in this child, early hypotonia and floppiness and abnormal eye movements precede the onset of hemiplegia, usually by several months. Frequent attacks of hemiplegia emerge as the predominant manifestation in the first decade. The episodes of hemiplegia last from minutes to days. The attacks can usually be aborted with sleep, and some parents report that they are increased by sleep deprivation. Cognitive delays become more severe with time. Between attacks the child is rarely normal. Persisting dyspraxia, dysarthria, dysphagia, dystonia, chorea, tremor, ataxia, weakness, and spasticity often occur. The swallowing difficulties are particularly concerning since aspiration pneumonia can occur.

Treatment of alternating hemiplegia of childhood has not been optimal. Sleep can relieve an attack. Benzodiazepines such as buccal midazolam have been used. Flunarizine, a drug that blocks calcium channels, has been widely used, although it does not stop acute attacks. The drug is rarely totally effective. Some reports suggest that it may be hazardous to withdraw flunarizine, in that the patient may suffer irreversible setbacks and exacerbations of spells following such a withdrawal.

> **KEY POINTS TO REMEMBER**
> - The duration of hemiplegia in the condition can vary considerably, lasting from seconds to hours.
> - Sleep relieves the symptoms.
> - A wide variety of neurological problems occur, including movement disorders such as dystonia.
> - Mutations in ATP1A3 are common but not uniform; other laboratory studies are primarily used to rule out other conditions.

Further Reading

Aicardi J, Bourgeois M, Goutières F. Alternating hemiplegia of childhood: clinical findings and diagnostic criteria. In: Andermann F, Aicardi J, Vigevano F, eds., *Alternating hemiplegia of childhood*. New York: Raven Press, 1995:3–18.

Mikati MA, Maguire H, Barlow CF, et al. A syndrome of autosomal dominant alternating hemiplegia: clinical presentation mimicking intractable epilepsy; chromosomal studies; and physiologic investigations. *Neurology* 1992;42:2257.

Neville BG, Ninan M. The treatment and management of alternating hemiplegia of childhood. *Dev Med Child Neurol* 2007;49:777–80.

Sakuragawa N. Alternating hemiplegia in childhood: 23 cases in Japan. *Brain Dev* 1992;14:283–8.

Sweeney MT, Newcomb TM, Swoboda KJ. The expanding spectrum of neurological phenotypes in children with ATP1A3 mutations, alternating hemiplegia of childhood, rapid-onset dystonia-Parkinsonism, CAPOS and beyond. *Pediatr Neurol* 2015;52:56–64.

Sweeney MT, Silver K, Gerard-Blanluet M, et al. Alternating hemiplegia of childhood: early characteristics and evolution of a neurodevelopmental syndrome. *Pediatrics* 2009;123:e534–41.

Viollet L, Glusman G, Murphy KJ, et al. Alternating hemiplegia of childhood: retrospective genetic study and genotype–phenotype correlations in 187 cubjects from the US AHCF registry. *PLoS One* 2015;10:e0127045; doi:10.1371/journal.pone.0127045

# 3 Newborn with a Rhythmic Twitch

You are called by the neonatologists in the neonatal intensive care unit to see a 7-day-old girl with apparent seizures. The child was born at term after an uneventful pregnancy, labor, and delivery. She was noted by the mother at age 6 days to have episodes where she would have bilateral jerks of the arms and legs. The jerks occurred in paroxysmal bursts lasting approximately 2 minutes. The child would flex the arms at the elbow and had rhythmic, to-and-fro movements of the forearms and legs. When informed of the events, the pediatrician told the mother to bring her daughter to the emergency room. There, the emergency room staff witnessed an event, concluded the child was having clonic seizures, administered a loading dose of phenobarbital (15 mg/kg), and admitted her to the hospital.

The child had electrolytes, glucose, CBC, calcium, magnesium, blood ammonia, liver function tests, a spinal fluid examination, and a head CT; all results were normal. Despite the phenobarbital, the child continued to have periodic episodes of myoclonic paroxysms. The child had an EEG and had an event of myoclonus during the recording. The neurologist reviewing the recording concluded that the myoclonic jerks were associated with theta and delta slowing with intermixed spikes. The child was then given a loading dose of phenytoin (15 mg/kg), still with no resolution of the myoclonus. The girl was then transported to your medical center. When you examine her you are pleased with how normal the child appears. She is alert and vigorous. The neurological examination is totally normal.

**What do you do now?**

## BENIGN NEONATAL SLEEP MYOCLONUS

Seizures in newborns are very serious events and often portend an ominous diagnosis and prognosis. While infants with normal neurological examinations can certainly have seizures, it is unusual to see this many seizures in an otherwise healthy newborn. After hearing the story, you question the mother about the events and whether these ever occurred when the child was awake with the eyes opened. The mother could not recall any events that occurred when the child was awake. The EEG from the referring hospital was reviewed and it was concluded that the record during and between myoclonic episodes was normal. The intermixed interictal spikes noted were thought to be artifact due to muscle activity during the events.

Based on the story and normal EEG, you conclude that the child has benign neonatal sleep myoclonus. You tell the neonatologists no further workup is warranted and discontinue the phenobarbital and phenytoin and discharge the child home. On follow-up 2 months later you learn that the girl no longer has myoclonus and is doing well developmentally.

Benign neonatal sleep myoclonus is characterized by myoclonic jerks in an otherwise healthy infant. The myoclonic jerks are usually bilaterally symmetrical with involvement of both the upper and lower extremities. The jerks are seen during sleep and are never present when the child is fully awake. Benign neonatal sleep myoclonus is a non-epileptic condition and is not associated with epileptiform discharges on the EEG. While the myoclonic jerks may be confused with clonic or myoclonic seizures, as shown in Table 3.1, there are distinguishing features that should lead to the correct diagnosis.

Benign neonatal sleep myoclonus occurs primarily in term, rather than preterm, infants. The onset of the myoclonus is very early, with the majority of the children having myoclonus during the first 2 weeks of life. All of the children outgrow their myoclonus and the developmental outlook is favorable.

Although the exact incidence of benign neonatal sleep myoclonus is not known, it does not appear to be a rare disorder. This condition has been well described in the literature, though it continues to be misdiagnosed by pediatricians, primary care physicians, and even pediatric neurologists. This misdiagnosis has often resulted in unnecessary diagnostic studies,

TABLE 3.1 **Benign Neonatal Sleep Myoclonus**

| Features | Clonic Seizures | Myoclonic Seizures | Benign Neonatal Sleep Myoclonus |
| --- | --- | --- | --- |
| Sleep state | Awake/sleep | Awake/sleep | Sleep |
| Movements | Clonic | Myoclonic | Myoclonic |
| Symmetry | Usually asymmetrical | Usually symmetrical | Usually symmetrical |
| Eyes | Open | Variable | Closed |
| EEG | Epileptiform discharges contralateral to side of body jerking | Markedly abnormal with generalized spike-wave | Normal, artifact is common |
| Response to antiepileptic drugs | Often effective | Moderately effective | Ineffective |

such as CT or MRI, and inappropriate antiepileptic drug therapy. The child presented here, for example, was subjected to radiation entailed by an unnecessary CT scan.

> **KEY POINTS TO REMEMBER**
> - Symmetrical irregular jerking of the upper and sometimes lower extremities
> - Myoclonic jerks can be quite dramatic.
> - Occurs only during sleep and ceases when the child is awakened
> - EEG is normal during the events.
> - No treatment is required.

Further Reading

Coulter DL, Allen RJ. Benign neonatal sleep myoclonus. *Arch Neurol* 1982;39:191–2.

di Capua M, Fusco L, Ricci S, et al. Benign neonatal sleep myoclonus: clinical features and video-polygraphic recordings. *Mov Disord* 1993;8:191–4.

Kaddurah AK, Holmes GL. Benign neonatal sleep myoclonus: history and semiology. *Pediatr Neurol* 2009;40:343–6.

Maurer VO, Rizzi M, Bianchetti MG, Ramelli GP. Benign neonatal sleep myoclonus: a review of the literature. *Pediatrics* 2010;125:e919–24.

Paro-Panjan D, Neubauer D. Benign neonatal sleep myoclonus: experience from the study of 38 infants. *Eur J Paediatr Neurol* 2008;12:14–8.

Ramelli GP, Sozzo AB, Vella S, et al. Benign neonatal sleep myoclonus: an under-recognized, non-epileptic condition. *Acta Paediatr* 2005;94:962–3.

# 4   Muteness at Breakfast

A pediatrician calls you about a 7-year-old boy he is seeing in his office. The parents brought the child in emergently because they thought he was having a stroke. That morning while eating breakfast the child suddenly stopped talking and developed a left facial droop and drooling. The parents said that when they asked the child what was wrong he did not respond but pointed to his mouth. The parents felt he understood the question but could not speak. The event lasted less than 5 minutes and cleared rapidly. When seen by his pediatrician he was normal.

When his pediatrician examines him he finds no neurological deficits. He tells you the child has a negative past medical history and family history. The pediatrician wonders if he should obtain an emergency head MRI.

You elect to see the child in clinic. On further questioning of the child you learn that he had tingling of his lips prior to tonic deviation of the lips. While the parents described a facial droop, what they actually were observing was positive motor activity with the lips pulled to the left. The child said he was aware of what was happening and knew what he wanted to say but could not speak. While as noted by the pediatrician the past medical history and neurological examination were unrevealing, the parents tell you he is struggling in the first grade. He has difficulty with language comprehension, speech articulation, and both auditory and visual memory.

**What do you do now?**

## BENIGN ROLANDIC EPILEPSY

This is a classic story for benign rolandic epilepsy (BRE), also known as benign epilepsy with centrotemporal spikes (BECTS). BECTS is a genetic disorder, confined to children, characterized by nocturnal focal or secondarily generalized seizures, and diurnal partial seizures arising from the lower rolandic area. The EEG pattern consists of midtemporal-central spike foci (Fig. 4–1). The disorder always begins during childhood, from 3 to 13 years, with a peak age of incidence between 7 and 8 years of life. The disorder occurs somewhat more frequently in boys than girls.

The additional history you heard from the child emphasizes the value of taking a history from your patients as well as their parents. The key features in this child were the motor impairment of the face and motor aphasia without impairment of consciousness. The observation that the child could understand the question yet could not speak is characteristic. As in this child, somatosensory symptoms may also occur, with the child noting tingling of the tongue, lips, and face during the initial phases of the

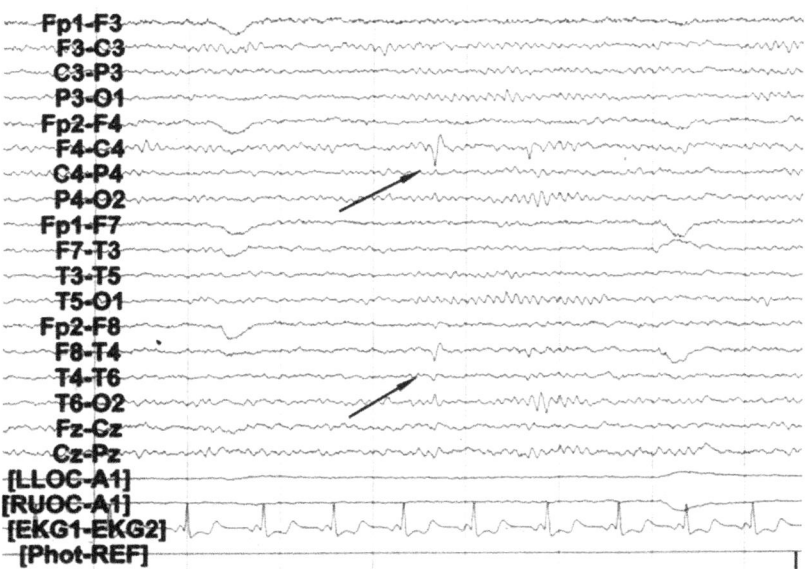

**FIGURE 4–1** Seven-year-old child with centrotemporal spikes (*arrows*) on the EEG. The child has benign rolandic epilepsy.

seizure. Some children have only diurnal simple partial seizures, whereas others have partial seizures with secondary generalization during sleep. In nocturnal seizures, the events typically feature clonic movements of the mouth with salivation and gurgling sounds from the throat. Secondary generalization of the nocturnal seizure is common. The initial focal component of the seizure may be quite brief and is often missed by the parents, who find the child in the midst of a generalized tonic-clonic seizure. Postictal confusion and amnesia are unusual after seizures in BRE.

The seizures may occur both during the day and during the night, although in most children, seizures are most common during sleep. Daytime and nocturnal seizures are both brief. The frequency of seizures in BRE is typically low, and status epilepticus is unusual.

If the patient's seizure history and EEG characteristics fit the BECTS profile and the normal neurological examination is normal, further workup is not necessary. If the neurological examination is abnormal or the EEG demonstrates abnormalities other than the typical epileptiform discharge, further evaluation with MRI is recommended.

Because of the benign nature of BRE, many physicians choose not to treat the first or second seizure. If treatment is initiated, the seizures are usually controlled with a single antiepileptic drug. Drugs used for partial seizures (e.g., levetiracetam, lamotrigine, phenobarbital, topiramate, carbamazepine, oxcarbazepine, or valproic acid) are usually effective. The EEG is not a good predictor of recurrence risk. Most patients can be tapered off medications after 1 to 2 years of seizure control, regardless of whether the EEG normalizes.

The prognosis of BRE is quite good, with almost all children going into remission by the teenage years. However, as with this child, a significant number of children with BRE have learning impairments with deficits in visual and auditory processing and memory and attention-deficit disorder. Children with BRE should be monitored closely for school performance. Fortunately, the learning difficulties typically abate once the seizures remit and the EEG normalizes.

The characteristic interictal EEG abnormality is a high-amplitude, usually diphasic spike with a prominent following slow wave. The spikes (<70 ms) or sharp waves (<200 ms) appear singly or in groups at the midtemporal (T3,T4) and central (rolandic) region (C3,C4). There is controversy as to whether the interictal spikes seen in BRE contribute to the cognitive impairment seen in many children. At the current time there is no evidence that trying to suppress epileptiform activity on the EEG improves outcome.

**KEY POINTS TO REMEMBER**

- Seizures during the day typically cause a motor aphasia without impairment of consciousness.
- Seizures occurring at night may be focal in onset and then evolve into a generalized convulsive seizure.
- Characteristic interictal spikes on EEG strongly support the diagnosis.
- Learning difficulties are common.
- The prognosis is excellent; antiepileptic drug therapy is usually not necessary.

Further Reading

Ambrosetto G, Tassinari CA. Antiepileptic drug treatment of benign childhood epilepsy with Rolandic spikes: Is it necessary? *Epilepsia* 1990;31:802–5.

Astradsson A, Olafsson E, Ludvigsson P, et al. Rolandic epilepsy: an incidence study in Iceland. *Epilepsia* 1998;39:884–6.

Camfield P, Camfield C. Epileptic syndromes in childhood: clinical features, outcomes, and treatment. *Epilepsia* 2002;43(Suppl 3):27–32.

Holmes GL. Clinical spectrum of benign focal epilepsies of childhood. *Epilepsia* 2000;41:1051–2.

Holmes GL. Rolandic epilepsy: clinical and electroencephalographic features. *Epilepsy Res* 1992(Suppl 6):29–43.

Kavros PM, Clarke T, Strug LJ, et al. Attention impairment in rolandic epilepsy: systematic review. *Epilepsia* 2008;49:1570–80.

Nicolai J, Aldenkamp AP, Arends J, et al. Cognitive and behavioral effects of nocturnal epileptiform discharges in children with benign childhood epilepsy with centrotemporal spikes. *Epilepsy Behav* 2006;8:56–70.

Northcott E, Connolly AM, Berroya A, et al. The neuropsychological and language profile of children with benign rolandic epilepsy. *Epilepsia* 2005;46:924–30.

Smith AB, Kavros PM, Clarke T, et al. A neurocognitive endophenotype associated with rolandic epilepsy. *Epilepsia* 2012;53:705–11.

van der Meij W, van Huffelen AC, Willemse J, et al. Rolandic spikes in the inter-ictal EEG of children: Contributions to diagnosis, classification and prognosis of epilepsy. *Dev Med Child Neurol* 1992;34:893–903.

# 5 Going Limp: A Case of Recurring Collapse

You receive a call from a nurse practitioner who wants you to see a boy with possible seizures. She tells you that this 16-month-old child has had multiple episodes where he loses consciousness and becomes quite limp and lifeless. The most recent episode progressed to a 30-second episode of tonic posturing with upgaze. After the first episode an EEG was obtained, which was normal. After the second episode the child was given phenobarbital, and a second EEG and an MRI of the brain (with sedation) were obtained. Both studies were normal. Despite a phenobarbital level of 30 µg/mL, the boy continues to have the episodes, which are very frightening to the parents.

When you see the boy you learn that he was developing normally until the onset of these spells. When you ask the mother to describe them she says the episodes always appear to begin with a temper tantrum, for example when the child hurts himself by falling, or when he does not get his way.

He cries for a few seconds and then passes out and turns blue. He is usually limp, but the mother noted that on one recent occasion he became rigid with upgaze. The child's eyes have otherwise always been closed during the episodes. When asked whether he ever had an attack that did not begin with crying the mother felt he may have done this once, although she is having difficulties remembering the details. He never has episodes when he is asleep. The mother remarked that since starting the phenobarbital the child has been irritable, with interrupted sleep, and has actually had more attacks.

### What do you do now?

## BREATH-HOLDING SPELLS/PALLID INFANTILE SYNCOPE

Based on the history alone you strongly suspect the child has breath-holding attacks. Since the child already had an EEG and MRI there is no need to repeat these studies, which might in retrospect have been obviated considering the history of precipitated spells of apparent syncope. Instead, you ask the mother to videotape one of the episodes and taper the child off the phenobarbital.

Breath-holding spells are very common in infants and young children. These are essentially episodes of syncope, precipitated by the combination of emotional upset and a deep inspiration. When they culminate in tonic posturing or a convulsion (i.e., convulsive syncope, which has no pathophysiologic connection to epilepsy), they may be mistaken for epileptic seizures. In rare cases, children may progress from benign, non-epileptic seizures in this setting to true and recurrent epileptic seizures, so-called anoxic reflexive epilepsy. These seizures may persist longer than non-epileptic convulsive syncope, which usually lasts less than a minute. Most frequently, the convulsive movements seen during breath-holding spells are reflex anoxic seizures and do not require antiepileptic drug therapy.

Although they are a benign disorder, as in this case, the attacks can be very frightening to the parents. Table 5.1 compares the salient features of breath-holding spells and pallid infantile syncope with the features of epileptic seizures. A key to breath-holding is that the spells usually begin with crying. However, in some children the trigger of crying can be quite brief, occurring after a sob or two, that may be overlooked by the observer. The child usually inspires and does not expire, may become cyanotic, falls down, and becomes limp. Unlike epileptic seizures, the eyes are typically closed during the syncopal attack, though there may be an upgaze in the case of a superimposed convulsion.

Pallid infantile syncope is precipitated by a stressful situation and leads to loss of consciousness. Pallor and sweating, as opposed to cyanosis, precede the loss of consciousness. The attacks occur in toddlers and can be precipitated by minor events such as blows to the head, fright, and frustration. In the past, the clinical diagnosis was confirmed in the EEG laboratory using controlled ocular compression while monitoring both the EEG

TABLE 5.1 **Breath-Holding Spells/Pallid Infantile Syncope**

| Clinical Features | Cyanotic Breath-Holding | Pallid Breath-Holding | Generalized Tonic or Tonic-Clonic Seizures |
|---|---|---|---|
| Age | 6 mo–6 yr | 12–18 mo | All ages |
| Precipitating factors | Invariably present | Invariably present | Usually none |
| Occurrence in sleep | Never | Never | Common |
| Family history | Often positive for breath-holding | Often positive for breath-holding | Often positive for seizures |
| Sequence of events | Crying → apnea → cyanosis → loss of consciousness → decreased tone → tonic-clonic or tonic seizure | Upset → pallor → loss of consciousness → hypotonia | Loss of consciousness → tonic-clonic or tonic seizure |
| Eyes open or closed | Closed | Closed | Open |
| Interictal EEG | Normal | Normal | Frequently abnormal |
| Postictal symptoms | Usually none | Usually none | Tired, confused, disoriented, sleepy |

and EKG; ocular compression would lead to severe bradycardia followed by asystole and EEG slowing. Because of a concern about retinal detachment as well as provoking a severe attack, this study is no longer done.

Although in this child an EEG and MRI were performed, with a typical history, these tests do not benefit the patient. Children with long QT syndrome have episodes of loss of consciousness that may be induced by injury, fright, or excitement, and an EKG should be obtained in a child with breath-holding or pallid infantile syncope. Since the condition appears to occur more frequently in children with iron deficiency anemia, obtaining a CBC and starting children with anemia on iron supplementation can be helpful. The prognosis is excellent, with the vast majority of children outgrowing the spells.

> **KEY POINTS TO REMEMBER**
> - Both cyanotic breath-holding spells and pallid infantile syncope are diagnosed by history.
> - Typically present in toddlers, or late in the first year of life, and remit after 3 to 4 years of age
> - Seizures (non-epileptic, convulsive syncope type) can occur during breath-holding attacks, but they should not be treated with antiepileptic drugs.
> - Treating children with breath-holding spells and iron deficiency anemia with iron supplementation can reduce the number of spells.
> - Obtain an EKG in patients with cyanotic breath-holding spells and pallid infantile syncope to rule out a prolonged QT interval.

Further Reading

Allsman L. Breath holding spells in children. *Adv Nurse Pract* 2008;16:53–4.

Arslan H, Torum E, Akkan JC, et al. The evaluation of physiological and biochemical parameters and the autonomic nervous systems of children with breath-holding spells. *Neuropediatrics* 2014;45:212–6.

DiMario FJ, Jr. Prospective study of children with cyanotic and pallid breath-holding spells. *Pediatrics* 2001;107:265–9.

DiMario FJ, Jr., Burleson JA. Behavior profile of children with severe breath-holding spells. *J Pediatr* 1993;122:488–491.

Holmes GL. Breath-holding attacks in children. *Postgrad Med* 1988;84:191–8.

Horrocks I, Nechay A, Stephenson JB, Zuberi SM. Anoxic-epileptic seizures: observational study of epileptic seizures induced by syncopes. *Arch Dis Child* 2005;90:1283–7.

Laxdal T, Gomez MR, Reiher J. Cyanotic and pallid syncopal attacks in children (breath-holding spells). *Dev Med Child Neurol* 1969;11:755–63.

Linder CW. Breath-holding spells in children. Studies of frequency, severity, management. *Clin Pediatr (Phila)* 1968;7:8–90.

Lombroso CT, Lerman P. Breath-holding spells (cyanotic and pallid infantile syncope). *Pediatrics* 1967;391:563–81.

Mocan H, Yildiran A, Orhan F, Erduran E. Breath holding spells in 91 children and response to treatment with iron. *Arch Dis Child* 1999;81:261–2.

Stephenson J. Anoxic-epileptic seizures: home video recordings of epileptic seizures induced by syncopes. *Epileptic Disord* 2004;6:15–9.

Stephenson JB. Clinical diagnosis of syncopes (including so-called breath-holding spells) without electroencephalography or ocular compression. *J Child Neurol* 2007;22:502–8.

Yilmaz S, Kukner S. Anemia in children with breath-holding spells. *J Pediatr* 1996;128:440–1.

# 6  Autonomic Storms En Route

You are asked to see an otherwise normal 6-year-old boy who had an unusual event while traveling in a car with his parents. The parents reported that he was quite happy and talkative on the trip until he complained that he was feeling sick. Within a minute he became quite pale and subdued. He gradually became more and more pale and kept complaining that he was going to vomit. He appeared restless and frightened. Within 10 minutes of the onset, his head and eyes slowly turned to the left. The eyes were opened but fixed in the left upper corner. At this point he was unresponsive. No convulsive activity was noted.

The parents explained: "We called his name but he was unresponsive. He had completely gone. We tried to move his head but it was fixed to the left." There were no convulsions. The event lasted for another 15 minutes. When his head and eyes returned to normal he looked better, although he was lethargic and confused. He then vomited profusely. When EMS arrived approximately 40 minutes from the onset of the episode he was still not aware of what was going on, although he was able to answer simple questions with yes or no. In the ER he slept for three-quarters of an hour and gradually came around, but it took him another hour to return to his baseline state.

When you see the patient an hour after he reached the ER he was quiet but answered questions appropriately. You learned from his parents that the child has been healthy except for several episodes of pronounced vomiting in the middle of the night. The family thought the child was confused and did not respond appropriately but attributed this to waking up suddenly from sleep. Your neurological examination is normal.

### What do you do now?

## PANAYIOTOPOULOS SYNDROME

This is a fairly classical story for Panayiotopoulos syndrome, a relatively common type of childhood epilepsy. While not as common as benign rolandic epilepsy, it occurs in approximately 10% of all cases of childhood epilepsy beginning earlier than the age of 6 years. The condition typically begins between 3 and 6 years of age, although many children have the condition earlier or later than the usual age range. Boys and girls appear to be equally affected and there does not appear to be a genetic predisposition.

The main seizure type is known as "autonomic." As in this child, there is often a sudden change in behavior and then the child becomes pale, complains of feeling sick, and usually vomits. The pupils typically dilate and there may be profuse sweating and drooling. Altered responsiveness typically ensues and may or may not be followed by tonic or tonic-clonic activity. Over two-thirds of the seizures occur in sleep, either during the night or during a daytime nap. The seizures are often quite long (20 to 60 minutes). Seizure frequency varies considerably, regardless of whether antiepileptic drugs are used. Some children will have only one seizure while others will have several per year.

The diagnosis of Panayiotopoulos syndrome is made based on a detailed account of the event. Important features in making the diagnosis are that the episodes often occur during sleep and are nearly always accompanied by autonomic features and vomiting. Age is also important as most seizures occur in preschool children. Since convulsive activity does not always occur it is likely that many children with the condition are undiagnosed.

You obtain an EEG and are told there are a few occipital sharp waves in the posterior head region. Unfortunately, the child did not sleep during the recording. This EEG finding would support the diagnosis of Panayiotopoulos syndrome. The EEG often shows paroxysmal activity (spikes and sharp waves) in the occipital region. However, the paroxysmal activity can be quite variable in regards to location, and in many children the EEG is normal.

Panayiotopoulos syndrome falls under the category of childhood epilepsies termed "benign epilepsy of childhood with occipital paroxysms" (BECOP). Panayiotopoulos syndrome is the early-onset type; the late-onset or Gastaut type consists of brief seizures with mainly visual symptoms such as elementary visual hallucinations, illusions, or amaurosis, followed by hemiclonic convulsions. Postictal migraine headaches are common in the Gastaut type. The interictal EEG in the Gastaut type is characterized by normal background activity and well-defined occipital discharges. The occipital discharges may be unilateral or bilateral and are increased during non–rapid eye movement sleep. An important feature in this syndrome is the prompt disappearance of EEG changes with eye opening and reappearance 1 to 20 seconds after eye closure. The prognosis in the late-onset (Gastaut) form is variable, with some children having seizures persisting into adulthood.

In this child neuroimaging is not necessary in view of the normal neurological examination. In children with nocturnal emesis, one must always be careful to be certain they do not have a posterior fossa brain tumor. With a normal examination a cerebellar or brainstem neoplasm would be quite unlikely.

Since the seizures happen infrequently and because most children will remit fairly quickly after onset, chronic antiepileptic drug therapy is usually not indicated. However, if the child has had three or more events and they are prolonged (lasting greater than 10 minutes), chronic antiepileptic drug therapy is indicated. There is no specific antiepileptic drug recommended, but in the United States, levetiracetam is most likely to be prescribed. Because prolonged seizures are common, parents should be given rescue medication (rectal diazepam) to abort the seizure if it lasts longer than 5 minutes.

### KEY POINTS TO REMEMBER

- Typically occurs in toddlers
- Nocturnal emesis is a common presenting feature.
- Seizures are either complex partial or generalized tonic-clonic.
- The EEG signature is occipital spikes, which typically are more common with eye closure.

Further Reading
Camfield P, Camfield C. Epileptic syndromes in childhood: clinical features, outcomes, and treatment. *Epilepsia* 2002;43(Suppl 3):27–32.

Caraballo R, Cersosimo R, Medina C, Fejerman N. Panayiotopoulos-type benign childhood occipital epilepsy: a prospective study. *Neurology* 2000;55:1096–100.

Covanis A. Panayiotopoulos syndrome: a benign childhood autonomic epilepsy frequently imitating encephalitis, syncope, migraine, sleep disorder, or gastroenteritis. *Pediatrics* 2006;118:e1237–43.

Panayiotopoulos CP. Benign childhood epilepsy with occipital paroxysms: a 15-year prospective study. *Ann Neurol* 1989;26:51–6.

Panayiotopoulos CP. Elementary visual hallucinations in migraine and epilepsy. *J Neurol Neurosurg Psychiat* 1994;57:1371–4.

Parisi P, Villa MP, Pelliccia A, et al. Panayiotopoulos syndrome: diagnosis and management. *Neurol Sci* 2007;28:72–79.

Schrader D, Shukla R, Gatrill R, et al. Epilepsy with occipital features in children: factors predicting seizure outcome and neuroimaging abnormalities. *Eur J Paediatr Neurol* 2011;15:15–20.

Taylor I, Berkovic SF, Kivity S, et al. Benign occipital epilepsies of childhood: clinical features and genetics. *Brain* 2008;131:2287–94.

# 7  A Frightful Awakening

You are called to the emergency room to see an 11-month-old boy who had a generalized tonic-clonic seizure. According to the parents, the child was doing well until the prior evening, when they said he felt hot and obtained an axillary temperature of 38.2°C. The boy was given 120 mg acetaminophen and was placed in the parents' bed. At approximately 3 a.m. the parents were awoken by the child kicking the mother. When the lights were turned on the parents found the child with the eyes open, staring straight ahead, with rhythmic jerking of the arms and legs. The family noted no color changes and estimated that the seizure lasted 5 minutes. The parents called 911 and the boy was transported to the hospital. The EMS personnel noted no seizures en route to the hospital.

On admission to the emergency room the child had a temperature of 38.5°C. The staff examined the boy and diagnosed acute otitis media. A spinal tap, which was normal, was performed and antibiotics and ibuprofen were started. CBC and electrolytes and glucose were normal. When you arrive, the boy is awake but is irritable. You learn from the parents that there is not a family history of epilepsy. The birth history was unrevealing and the child's development has been normal. Your examination is unremarkable.

The emergency room staff has made arrangements to obtain a CT scan of the head and ask you whether it would be better to do an MRI.

**What do you do now?**

## FEBRILE SEIZURES

By the presentation, this boy had a simple febrile seizure. The seizure occurred in a child between 3 months and 5 years of age, was associated with fever, was generalized tonic-clonic in type, and lasted less than 15 minutes. With a normal neurological examination there is little reason to do any additional workup, and you should tell the staff that neither the CT nor MRI is necessary.

The most important test done when the child arrived in the emergency room was the spinal tap. While not all children with febrile seizures need to be tapped, the American Academy of Pediatrics recommends, on the basis of the published evidence and consensus, that after the first seizure with fever in infants younger than 12 months, a lumbar puncture be strongly considered because the clinical signs and symptoms associated with meningitis may be minimal. While clinical judgment is paramount, missing meningitis can be deadly and it is better to be cautious. The American Academy of Pediatrics also does not recommend the routine drawing of serum electrolytes, calcium, phosphorus, magnesium, CBC, or blood glucose. In this case, having a serum glucose to compare with the cerebrospinal glucose would be useful, particularly if the spinal fluid glucose was low, as can be seen in children with glucose transporter deficiencies. Furthermore, EEG and neuroimaging should not be done based on the history and neurological examination.

While additional testing is not necessary, it is important to counsel the family. While the risk of developing epilepsy after a simple febrile seizure is low, there is a substantial risk that the child will have another febrile seizure. As long as the seizures are brief and nonfocal and associated with fever, it is not necessary to bring the child into the hospital. However, the cause of the fever should be investigated by the pediatrician.

Children who have focal seizures, prolonged febrile seizures, or more than one in 24 hours have a higher likelihood of developing epilepsy. Whether febrile status epilepticus (a seizure lasting more than 30 minutes in which the only etiology is fever) causes damage that leads to subsequent temporal lobe epilepsy or whether febrile status epilepticus is due to an abnormal brain to begin with remains controversial. However, recent studies of febrile status epilepticus have shown that a proportion of the children will have signal abnormalities and swelling in the temporal lobe that over time lead to hippocampal sclerosis.

Febrile seizures are rarely treated since for the most part they are quite benign and all of the antiepileptic drugs have some side effects. However, when children have prolonged febrile seizures, rectal diazepam can be used to abort the seizure.

> **KEY POINTS TO REMEMBER**
>
> - When evaluating a child with a seizure occurring during a febrile illness, it is essential to consider the possibility of an intracranial infection.
> - The only diagnostic test to be considered when evaluating a child with a simple febrile seizure is an examination of the cerebrospinal fluid.
> - Antiepileptic drug therapy is not indicated in children with febrile seizures.
> - Consider rectal diazepam for children with prolonged febrile seizures (more than 5 minutes).

Further Reading

American Academy of Pediatrics, Committee on Quality Improvement, Subcommittee on Febrile Seizures. Practice parameter: Long-term treatment of the child with simple febrile seizures. *Pediatrics* 1999;103:1307–9.

Annegers JF, Blakley SA, Hauser WA, Kurland LT. Recurrence of febrile convulsions in a population-based cohort. *Epilepsy Res* 1990;5:209–16.

Hesdorffer DC, Shinnar S, Lewis DV, et al. Risk factors for febrile status epilepticus: a case-control study. *J Pediatr* 2013;163:1147–51.

Hirtz DG, Camfield CS, Camfield PR. Febrile convulsions. In: Engel J Jr, Pedley TA, eds., *Epilepsy: a comprehensive textbook*. Philadelphia: Lippincott-Raven, 1997:2483–8.

Lewis DV, Shinnar S, Hesdorffer DC, et al. Hippocampal sclerosis after febrile status epilepticus: the FEBSTAT study. *Ann Neurol* 2014;75:178–85.

Nelson KB, Ellenberg JH. Predictors of epilepsy in children who have experienced febrile seizures. *N Engl J Med* 1976;295:1029–33.

Nelson KB, Ellenberg JH. Prognosis in children with febrile seizures. *Pediatrics* 1978;61:720–727.

Patterson KP, Baram TZ, Shinnar S. Origins of temporal lobe epilepsy: febrile seizures and febrile status epilepticus. *Neurotherapeutics* 2014;11:242–50.

Seinfeld S, Shinnar S, Sun S, et al. Emergency management of febrile status epilepticus: results of the FEBSTAT study. *Epilepsia* 2014;55:388–95.

Sillanpaa M, Camfield P, Camfield C, et al. Incidence of febrile seizures in Finland: prospective population-based study. *Pediatr Neurol* 2008;38:391–4.

# 8 Beyond Colic: The Distant Infant

You are called to the emergency room about a 9-month-old girl who was brought to the hospital because of peculiar spells characterized by sudden flexion of the trunk and extension of the arms. The family says the spells have been going on for approximately 3 weeks. They are brief, lasting less than 5 seconds, but occur in flurries, with 10 to 15 spells occurring in sequence. The parents state the episodes often occur upon awakening. Further questioning by the emergency room staff revealed that since the spells began, the girl has been less interactive and no longer smiles or follows with her eyes. The family says the pediatrician believes the child is having colic and came to the emergency room because they are concerned that she has something more ominous.

You tell the emergency room staff to arrange for an EEG and a visit with you in your office the next day. When the girl arrives you learn that she was delivered after a normal pregnancy and labor. Birth weight and Apgar scores were normal and the child was discharged from the hospital on the second day of life.

Early developmental milestones were normal. By age 6 months the child was sitting, reaching for toys, transferring objects between hands, and rolling over and supported weight when held upright. The parents tell you she was quite sociable, squealed when happy, babbled chains of consonants, and responded to her name. However, when she began having the so-called colic spells there was a dramatic change in her alertness and activity level: she no longer showed interest in people and toys, stopped smiling and babbling, and often seemed distant. The girl also had episodes of severe irritability that would occur without provocation and sometimes would last an hour or more. The parents were quite skeptical about the diagnosis of colic and felt the girl had a serious problem.

The episodes of trunk flexion and extension of the arms occurred multiple times daily. Each episode consisted of 6 to 12 spasms. All of the events were similar in their behavioral features.

On examination you find a child who lies rather passively and did not interact with either you or the parents. She had a normal head circumference. She would not follow, but did look about the room. Funduscopic examination was normal. The tone was decreased and the reflexes were symmetrical. The child sat without support and had good head control in the sitting position.

The EEG done before the girl's clinical visit was quite abnormal, showing hypsarrhythmia. Several spasms were recorded during the EEG. The EEG during the spasm showed a high-amplitude, sharply contoured delta wave at the vertex followed by a decremental pattern.

### What do you do now?

## INFANTILE SPASMS

After a review of the EEG you go back to the clinic and ask the parents to remove the child's clothes. On close examination you note that there are multiple hypopigmented macules.

The emergency room staff is describing typical infantile spasms, a unique and malignant epileptic syndrome confined to infants. The characteristic features of this syndrome are tonic or myoclonic seizures, hypsarrhythmic EEGs, and mental retardation; the triad of infantile spasms, hypsarrhythmic EEGs, and mental retardation is referred to as West's syndrome. Not all infants with infantile spasms conform strictly to this definition. The disorder is also referred to in the literature as massive spasms, salaam seizures, flexion or flexor spasms, jackknife seizures, and massive myoclonic jerks.

Infantile spasms are an age-specific disorder beginning in children during the first 2 years of life. The peak age of onset is 4 to 6 months of age. Approximately 90% of infantile spasms begin before 12 months of age. It is rare for them to begin during the first 2 weeks of life or after 18 months.

The parents were correct to be concerned that the child has something more serious than colic. The syndrome of infantile spasms is rightfully considered to be a medical emergency, not because the spasms are life-threatening but because they are frequently associated with developmental arrest or regression. Some studies have shown that children who are diagnosed and treated early, within days or weeks of the diagnosis, fare better than those in which the diagnosis is delayed.

While the diagnosis can typically be made based on the history, having the parents make a videotape of the events can be very helpful in establishing the diagnosis. While gastrointestinal reflux could conceivably be confused with infantile spasms, children with reflux typically do not have repetitive episodes of tonic or myoclonic events.

If infantile spasms are suspected, the child should have an EEG. Infantile spasms are usually associated with markedly abnormal EEGs. The most commonly found EEG pattern is hypsarrhythmia (Fig. 8–1). This pattern consists of high-amplitude slow waves mixed with spikes and sharp waves whose amplitude and topography vary in an asynchronous manner

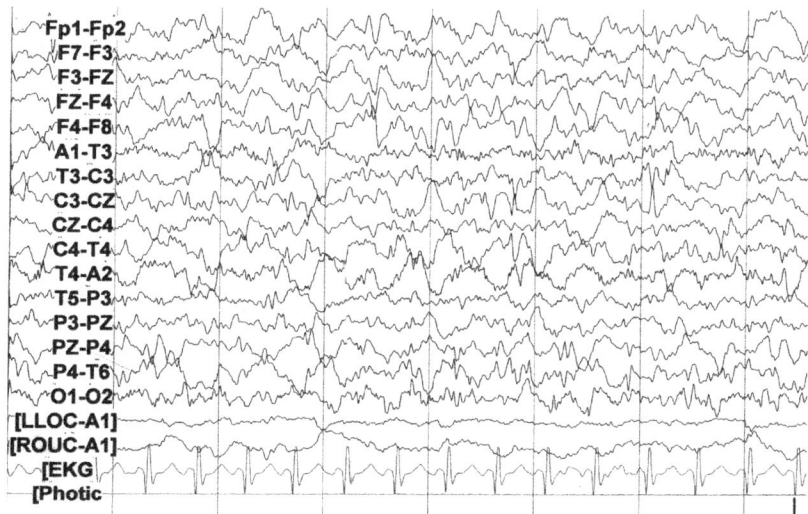

**FIGURE 8-1** Hypsarrhythmia pattern in a 9-month-old with infantile spasms. Note the high-voltage chaotic pattern with multifocal spikes and sharp waves.

between the two hemispheres. The background activity is completely disorganized and chaotic. During sleep, there are bursts of polyspike and slow waves. Somewhat surprising, in view of the marked background abnormalities, is the presence of sleep spindles in some patients. During rapid eye movement sleep there may be a marked diminution or complete disappearance of the hypsarrhythmic pattern.

Once the diagnosis is established, the child needs to be evaluated for the etiology of infantile spasms and started on therapy. In this case the MRI showed periventricular and cortical tubers (Fig. 8–2). These findings, in conjunction with the hypopigmented macules on the child's skin, would establish the diagnosis of tuberous sclerosis. Infantile spasms are treated with adrenocorticotropic hormone (ACTH) or vigabatrin. Children with tuberous sclerosis as a cause of the infantile spasms appear to respond better to vigabatrin than children with other causes of the spasms.

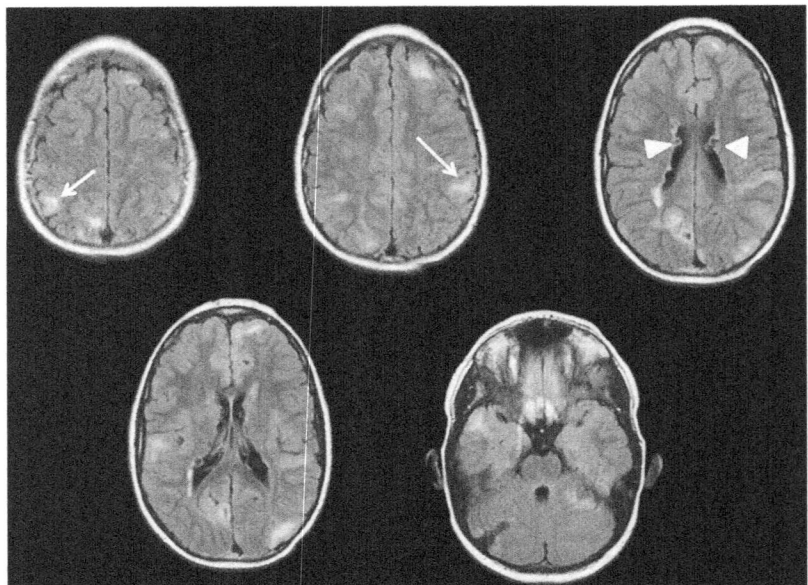

**FIGURE 8-2** MRI showing subependymal nodules (*arrowheads*) and cortical tubers (*arrows*).

> **KEY POINTS TO REMEMBER**
> - Age-related seizures beginning in the first year of life
> - Child has flurries of flexor, extensor, or mixed tonic seizures
>   The EEG is critical to the diagnosis, showing markedly abnormal patterns such as hypsarrhythmia.
> - A normal EEG during waking and sleep would make the diagnosis unlikely.
> - Determining the etiology of spasms is critical in determining the child's prognosis.

Further Reading

Dimassi S, Labalme A, Ville D, et al. Whole-exome sequencing improves the diagnosis yield in sporadic infantile spasm syndrome. *Clin Genet* 2015 Jul 3 [Epub ahead of print].

Epi4K Consortium. De novo mutations in epileptic encephalopathies. *Nature* 2013;501:217–221.

Goh S, Kwiatkowski DJ, Dorer DJ, Thiele EA. Infantile spasms and intellectual outcomes in children with tuberous sclerosis complex. *Neurology* 2005;65:235–8.

Hancock E, Osborne J, Milner P. Treatment of infantile spasms. *Cochrane Database Syst Rev* 2003;CD001770.

Hrachovy RA, Frost JD Jr., Kellaway P. Hypsarrhythmia: variations on the theme. *Epilepsia* 1984;25:317–25.

Lux AL, Edwards SW, Hancock E, et al. The United Kingdom Infantile Spasms Study (UKISS) comparing hormone treatment with vigabatrin on developmental and epilepsy outcomes to age 14 months: a multicentre randomised trial. *Lancet Neurol* 2005;4:712–27.

Lux AL, Edwards SW, Hancock E, et al. The United Kingdom Infantile Spasms Study comparing vigabatrin with prednisolone or tetracosactide at 14 days: a multicentre, randomised controlled trial. *Lancet* 2004;364:1773–8.

Lux AL, Osborne JP. The influence of etiology upon ictal semiology, treatment decisions and long-term outcomes in infantile spasms and West syndrome. *Epilepsy Res* 2006;70(Suppl 1):S77–86.

Mackay MT, Weiss SK, Adams-Webber T, et al. Practice parameter: medical treatment of infantile spasms: report of the American Academy of Neurology and the Child Neurology Society. *Neurology* 2004;62:1668–81.

Vigevano F, Fusco L, Pachatz C. Neurophysiology of spasms. *Brain Dev* 2001;23:467–72.

# 9 The Twitch That Came Before

You get a call from a local emergency room about a 14-year-old girl whose mother found her in bed at 6 a.m. having a generalized tonic-clonic seizure. The duration of the seizure was unknown. When seen in the ER she was postictal but had an otherwise normal neurological examination. Workup in the ER revealed a normal CT scan, CBC, electrolytes, and liver function tests. The patient and her mother denied any prior seizures.

You recommend that she make an appointment with you for an outpatient visit and suggest holding treatment at this time. She tells you that she has been under a great deal of stress recently, having broken up with a boyfriend. She does not sleep well and had difficulty falling asleep the night before the seizure. Despite the negative history given by the patient and her mother in the ER about prior seizures, you ask about possible jerks of her hands, particularly in the morning.

The patient tells you that on some mornings, she is somewhat tremulous and has had some twitching of her hands on occasion.

Her neurological examination is normal and the family history is negative.

**What do you do now?**

## JUVENILE MYOCLONIC EPILEPSY

Considering the age of onset (early teenage years), timing (early morning), provoking factors (sleep deprivation), and history of probable myoclonic jerks, the most likely diagnosis is juvenile myoclonic epilepsy (JME).

You decide to do an EEG, instructing the patient to retire late at night and wake up early in the morning so that she will sleep during the recording. The EEG showed a normal background pattern for age, with 9-Hz alpha rhythm along with normal sleep features (symmetrical sleep spindles and vertex sharp waves). Intermittent bursts of generalized, fast spike-and-wave activity of 4 Hz lasting less than 3 seconds were seen. These generalized discharges were more frequent during drowsiness and sleep. Photic stimulation and hyperventilation failed to elicit any discharges.

The EEG supports the diagnosis of JME, and you decide to start the patient on levetiracetam, starting at 500 mg bid and increasing to 1,000 mg bid. You also start her on clonazepam dissolvable tablets (0.5 mg), as needed, for flurries of myoclonic seizures.

JME is a familial disorder that typically begins in the second decade of life and is characterized by mild myoclonic seizures, generalized tonic-clonic or clonic-tonic-clonic seizures (a variation of generalized tonic-clonic seizures in which there is an initial clonic or myoclonic phase), and occasionally absence seizures. The myoclonic seizures are usually mild to moderate in intensity and involve the neck, shoulders, and arms. They can occur either singly or repetitively and may cause the patient to drop objects.

Rarely, the jerks may involve the legs and cause the patient to fall to the ground. There have been multiple attempts at determining the gene or genes responsible for the disorder. It now appears that there is not a single gene that accounts for all of the cases and that there is considerable genetic and locus heterogeneity in the disorder.

The interictal EEG in this disorder is distinctive and easily distinguished from other forms of generalized epilepsies. The characteristic feature of the EEG is the fast (3.5- to 6-Hz) spike-and-wave and multiple spike-and-wave complexes (Fig. 9–1). This pattern contrasts with the 3-Hz spike-and-wave complexes seen in classic absence seizures (Fig. 9–2) and the slow (1.5- to 2.5-Hz) spike-and-wave complexes of the Lennox-Gastaut syndrome (Fig. 9–3).

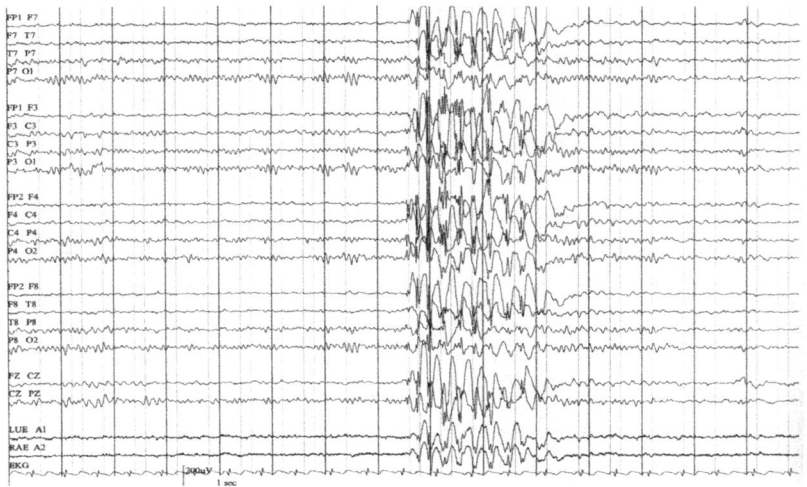

**FIGURE 9-1** Rapid spike-wave discharge in a 14-year-old girl with juvenile myoclonic epilepsy.

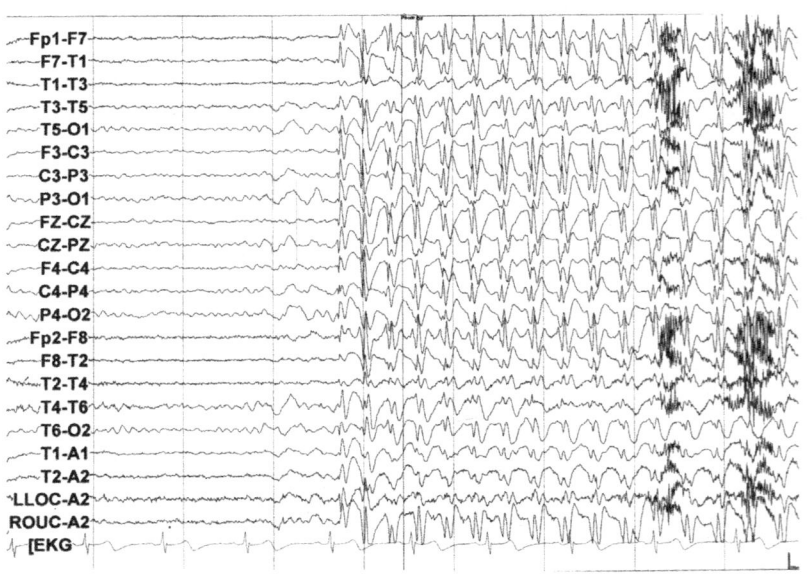

**FIGURE 9-2** 3-Hz spike-wave from a 6-year-old with typical absence seizure.

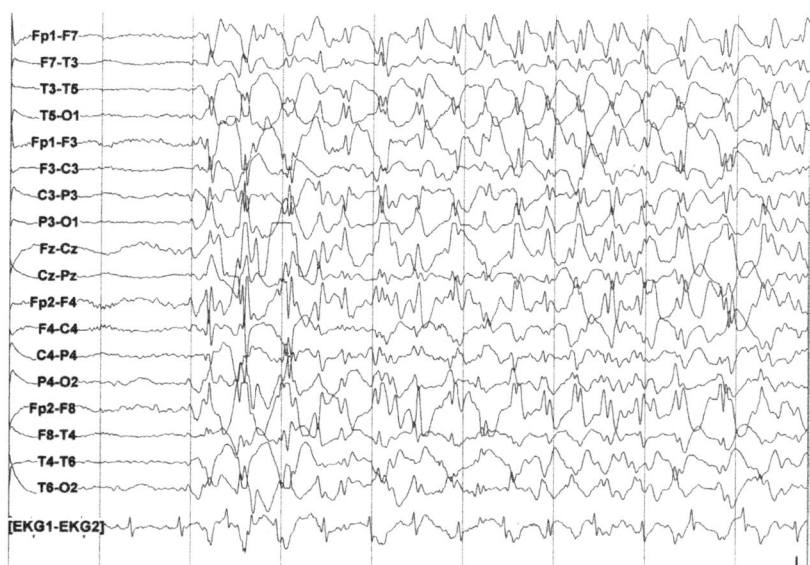

**FIGURE 9-3** Slow spike-wave from a 12-year-old with Lennox-Gastaut syndrome.

JME falls within the category of idiopathic generalized epilepsies, which account for approximately 15% to 20% of all epilepsies. The seizure types are typical absence seizures, myoclonic jerks, and generalized tonic-clonic seizures, alone or in varying combinations and with variable severity. The seizures tend to be more frequent on awakening and with sleep deprivation. In addition to JME, other epilepsy syndromes of adolescence include juvenile absence epilepsy, idiopathic generalized epilepsy with tonic-clonic seizures, and grand mal on awakening. The classification of idiopathic generalized epilepsies follows two schools of thought; one maintains that the various types constitute different and separate syndromes, while the other suggests that the idiopathic generalized epilepsies are one biological continuum.

In a patient with a normal neurological examination and a history and EEG compatible with JME, neuroimaging (CT or MRI) is not necessary. However, most patients who have a generalized tonic-clonic seizure will have a CT or MRI in the emergency room. While from a medical standpoint such scanning is of little value, a normal neuroimaging study in a teenager with generalized tonic-clonic seizures can be reassuring to both the family and physician.

In this case the patient was started on treatment after a single generalized tonic-clonic seizure. As a rule, patients with a single seizure are not placed on chronic antiepileptic drug therapy. However, in this case the teenager already had a history of myoclonic seizures.

Drugs that are often effective in this condition include valproate, levetiracetam, and lamotrigine. Valproate and levetiracetam are effective in both the generalized tonic-clonic and myoclonic seizures, whereas the efficacy of lamotrigine in myoclonic seizures is more variable. Clonazepam can be quite useful for the myoclonic jerks.

As important as the drug therapy is the counseling that should occur at the first visit. It is important for the patient to be compliant with antiepileptic drug therapy and to avoid sleep deprivation and heavy alcohol consumption. Explaining to the patient that sleep deprivation is used to increase epileptiform discharges on the EEG often brings home the message that adequate sleep will reduce the likelihood of a seizure.

While at one time JME was considered a lifelong disorder, it is now known that approximately 20% of the patients will eventually go into remission and come off antiepileptic drugs. The majority of patients respond well to antiepileptic drug therapy. Unfortunately, 75% of patients with JME have depression and unfavorable social outcomes, including social isolation, unemployment, and social impulsiveness, complicating the lives of many patients.

---

**KEY POINTS TO REMEMBER**

- Typically starts in adolescence
- Patients may not be aware they are having myoclonic seizures since they can be quite mild and be considered a nuisance rather than a serious problem.
- The EEG shows rapid spike-and-wave discharges. However, the discharges can be infrequent, and a normal EEG does not rule out the condition.
- While patients typically respond well to antiepileptic therapy, the condition usually is lifelong.

Further Reading

Asconapé J, Penry JK. Some clinical and EEG aspects of benign juvenile myoclonic epilepsy. *Epilepsia* 1984;25:108–14.

Baykan B, Martinez-Juarez IE, Altindag EA, et al. Lifetime prognosis of juvenile myoclonic epilepsy. *Epilepsy Behav* 2013;28(Suppl 1):S18–24.

Beghi M, Beghi E, Cornaggia CM, Gobbi G. Idiopathic generalized epilepsies of adolescence. *Epilepsia* 2006;47(Suppl 2):107–10.

Camfield C, Camfield P. Management guidelines for children with idiopathic generalized epilepsy. *Epilepsia* 2005;46(Suppl 9):112–6.

Camfield CS, Camfield PR. Juvenile myoclonic epilepsy 25 years after seizure onset: a population-based study. *Neurology* 2009;73:1041–5.

Delgado-Escueta AV, Enrile-Bascal FE. Juvenile myoclonic epilepsy of Janz. *Neurology* 1984;34:285–94.

Koepp MJ, Thomas RH, Wandschneider B, et al. Concepts and controversies of juvenile myoclonic epilepsy: still an enigmatic epilepsy. *Expert Rev Neurother* 2014;14:819–31.

Panayiotopolous CP, Obeid T, Tahan AR. Juvenile myoclonic epilepsy: a 5-year prospective. *Epilepsia* 1994;35:285–96.

Wirrell EC, Camfield CS, Camfield PR, et al. Long-term prognosis of typical childhood absence epilepsy: remission or progression to juvenile myoclonic epilepsy. *Neurology* 1996;47:912–8.

# 10 Airway, Breathing, Circulation, and Anticonvulsants

You are called to the emergency room to see a 6-year-old boy. The child has epilepsy likely due to a hypoxic-ischemic injury at birth. He has been having one or two generalized tonic-clonic seizures per month and has been taking carbamazepine and valproic acid. On the day of admission he apparently was doing well until he had a generalized tonic-clonic seizure that persisted despite rectal diazepam (7.5 mg). He was taken to the emergency room and continued to have the seizure despite another dose of diazepam (7.5 mg) intravenously. The emergency room staff says the seizure has lasted approximately 45 minutes. He is estimated to weigh 22 kg.

**What do you do now?**

## STATUS EPILEPTICUS

Generalized Status epilepticus is a condition in which the seizure lasts 30 minutes or more without any period during which the child regains consciousness. This is a medical emergency that requires prompt intervention. Priorities begin with ABC's—ensure an open airway and adequate oxygenation. Reliable intravenous access is necessary. The blood pressure should be monitored and adequate glucose levels maintained. If the child appears hypoxic (cyanotic) or to be hypoventilating, he or she should be intubated.

The longer the seizure continues, the more difficult it is to stop, so that aggressive management with intravenous medication is necessary. A progressive reduction of surface expression of GABA(A) receptors, due to intracellular accumulation of the receptors, likely contributes to the reduced effectiveness of benzodiazepines. In addition, accumulation of extracellular potassium and intracellular calcium at the synapse contribute to heightened excitability. Your primary advice is to further intensify the anticonvulsant medications.

While diazepam is widely used for status epilepticus, the child did not respond to two doses. Lorazepam (0.1–0.15 mg/kg) is a first-line drug for status due to its longer distribution half-life than diazepam, which results in a lower incidence of status epilepticus recurrence. In clinical trials lorazepam appears to be superior to other drugs. Therefore, despite the failure of diazepam, a dose of lorazepam should be the first step.

If lorazepam was not effective, you should treat with intravenous levetiracetam (20 mg/kg). If levetiracetam was not effective, fosphenytoin (15–20 mg/kg of phenytoin equivalents) should be given. (If there were an inadvertent extravasation of the drug, fosphenytoin would be less likely than phenytoin to cause venous sclerosis, the "purple glove" syndrome.) Each trial should be given about 15 minutes before transitioning to the next trial.

If fosphenytoin was not effective, intravenous phenobarbital (15–20 mg/kg) could be used. At this point the child should be intubated and should be in the intensive care unit, since phenobarbital in combination with a benzodiazepine could lead to respiratory depression. Phenobarbital produces considerable sedation, making it difficult to monitor neurological function after the status epilepticus has ceased. Valproic acid (20–25 mg/kg) has been used for status epilepticus, although there are concerns about valproic acid–induced liver toxicity.

If fosphenytoin was not effective you could use a continuous infusion of midazolam, a benzodiazepine, or pentobarbital, a barbiturate. The goal of midazolam or pentobarbital is to put the EEG into burst suppression in order to disrupt the continuous seizure activity, allowing the brain to recover. Table 10.1 provides a summary of antiepileptic drugs used to treat status epilepticus.

Children with status epilepticus should have continuous EEG monitoring. This is critical if the child is given a paralytic agent, since ongoing status epilepticus can be detrimental even when pharmacological paralysis stops the outward seizure activity. In this setting, EEG monitoring permits assessment of the effectiveness of the midazolam or pentobarbital.

Concurrent to targeting the status epilepticus, the physician will want to consider precipitating factors for the status epilepticus. In a child with known epilepsy, one of the more commonly identified causes would be nonadherence to the prescribed antiepileptic drugs. Serum levels of carbamazepine and valproic acid will be important. The etiologies of status epilepticus are in general as varied as those of epilepsy in general. Most cases have a symptomatic etiology, although idiopathic cases can occur.

TABLE 10.1 **Drugs Used to Treat Status Epilepticus**

| Drug | Intravenous Dosage |
| --- | --- |
| Diazepam | 0.3–0.5 mg/kg (rectal or intravenous) |
| Lorazepam | 0.1–0.15 mg/kg |
| Levetiracetam | 20 mg/kg |
| Fosphenytoin | 15–20 mg/kg phenytoin equivalents |
| Phenobarbital | 15–20 mg/kg |
| Valproate | 20–25 mg/kg |
| Midazolam | 0.15-mg/kg bolus followed by a 1- to 5-µg/kg/min infusion |
| Pentobarbital | 5-mg/kg loading dose, then a 1- to 3-mg/kg/hr continuous infusion |

Acute precipitants are distinguished from ultimate causes of status epilepticus. The former include nonspecific febrile illness, rapid drug withdrawal, trauma, and toxins. The latter include hypoxic-ischemic encephalopathy, infection, or the occurrence of status epilepticus as a manifestation of the primary epilepsy syndrome. The etiology of the status epilepticus is the major determinant of the outcome.

> **KEY POINTS TO REMEMBER**
> - The longer status epilepticus persists, the more difficult it will be to stop.
> - The airway must be protected and venous access must be achieved.
> - Lorazepam is a first-line therapy for status epilepticus.
> - The etiology of the status epilepticus is critical, since it is the primary factor in determining the outcome.

Further Reading

Abend NS, Monk HM, Licht DJ, Dlugos DJ. Intravenous levetiracetam in critically ill children with status epilepticus or acute repetitive seizures. *Pediatr Crit Care Med* 2009;10:505–10.

Chin RF, Neville BG, Peckham C, Bedford H, et al. Incidence, cause, and short-term outcome of convulsive status epilepticus in childhood: prospective population-based study. *Lancet* 2006;368:222–9.

Goodkin HP, Yeh JL, Kapur J. Status epilepticus increases the intracellular accumulation of GABAA receptors. *J Neurosci* 2005;25:5511–20.

Goodkin HR, Joshi S, Kozhemyakin M, Kapur J. Impact of receptor changes on treatment of status epilepticus. *Epilepsia* 2007;48(Suppl 8):14–5.

Hussain N, Appleton R, Thorburn K. Aetiology, course and outcome of children admitted to paediatric intensive care with convulsive status epilepticus: a retrospective 5-year review. *Seizure* 2007;16:305–12.

Khongkhatithum C, Thampratankul L, Wiwattanadittakul N, Visudtibhan A. Intravenous levetiracetam in Thai children and adolescents with status epilepticus and acute repetitive seizures. *Eur J Paediatr Neurol* 2015;19:429–34.

Neville BG, Chin RF, Scott RC. Childhood convulsive status epilepticus: epidemiology, management and outcome. *Acta Neurol Scand Suppl* 2007;186:21–4.

Raspall-Chaure M, Chin RF, Neville BG, Bedford H, Scott RC. The epidemiology of convulsive status epilepticus in children: a critical review. *Epilepsia* 2007;48:1652–63.

Riviello JJ, Jr., Ashwal S, Hirtz D, et al. Practice parameter: diagnostic assessment of the child with status epilepticus (an evidence-based review): report of the Quality Standards Subcommittee of the American Academy of Neurology and the Practice Committee of the Child Neurology Society. *Neurology* 2006;67:1542–50.

Riviello JJ, Jr., Holmes GL. The treatment of status epilepticus. *Semin Pediatr Neurol* 2004;11:129–38.

Scott RC, Kirkham FJ. Clinical update: childhood convulsive status epilepticus. *Lancet* 2007;370:724–6.

# SECTION II

# Congenital and Genetic Disorders

## 11 A Question of Family History

A 3-year-old boy is brought in by his father because of a concern of possible hereditary neuropathy. This concern arises because the mother, who has been estranged from the family for more than 2 years, carried a diagnosis of some type of hereditary neuropathy, with others of her immediate family members also affected: her brother, mother, and maternal grandmother. The father of your patient knows little else about the family history, or their diagnosis, but he is aware that the mother had some mild generalized weakness: she was a relatively slow runner and stair climber, and had complained of always having a relatively weak grip when it came to removing jar lids and so forth. On examination, the child seems to have good strength and running gait and normal cranial nerves and sensory testing. Indeed, his examination seems entirely normal, but it is difficult to elicit his ankle jerk reflexes.

**What do you do now?**

## CHARCOT MARIE TOOTH

There is a compelling case here that this patient has a neurological problem based on family history and the absence of ankle jerk reflexes, which is decidedly abnormal at this age. The most likely diagnosis appears to be one of several different subtypes of hereditary neuropathy with either X-linked or autosomal dominant inheritance: the pedigree virtually excludes recessive inheritance, and the absence of father-to-son transmission opens the possibility of X-linked inheritance. As a group, Charcot Marie Tooth (CMT) disorders, also known as hereditary motor sensory neuropathies, represent the most common hereditary degenerative conditions of the nervous system. Featuring diverse inheritance patterns, they have been associated with over 60 different genes.

At this point, the main tests to consider would include electrophysiological testing (electromyography, nerve conduction velocity) and genetic testing. The value of electrophysiological testing is that it can help confirm the expected findings of a genetically based polyneuropathy (there should be some in the face of ankle hyporeflexia) and can further localize the lesion as either an axonopathy (decreased amplitudes) or a demyelinative process (slowed conduction velocities). It should also be noted that the sensitivity of the genetic testing in this setting is itself a fairly complex question since there are several possibilities for underlying types of familial neuropathy and associated genetic mutations, as outlined in Table 11.1.

In general, about 80% of hereditary motor sensory neuropathy cases are of the demyelinating type and can be identified as having an underlying mutation in either PMP22, MPZ, MFN2, or GJB1. CMTX (type 1—there are several other subtypes) is said to be the second most common type after CMT1a (PMP22).

In this case, considering that the patient is in effect presymptomatic, arriving at a specific genetic diagnosis carries no significant therapeutic contingency for the patient. There appears to be no practical gain from either electrophysiological or genetic testing at this juncture. You advise the parent of the suspected diagnosis. Though he presses for further testing now "just to be sure," he ultimately agrees to defer the test, leaving reluctantly.

TABLE 11.1  **Some Types of Familial Neuropathy and Associated Genetic Mutations***

| Neuropathy Rubric | Neuropathology | Genetic Tests* |
| --- | --- | --- |
| CMT1 | Schwann cell (demyelinating) | PMP22 |
| CMT2 | Axon | Numerous |
| CMT-X | Mixed axonal/demyelinating | GJB1 (connexin 32) |

*In some cases, the sensitivity of the genetic test for the given condition has not been established—remember that these tests are in general more useful for "ruling in" than "ruling out" any of the conditions.

The child is lost to follow-up but returns at age 12 because, following a concussion, he underwent a head MRI and was found to have a large, unifocal, T2 bright area in the right centrum semi-ovale. During the intervening 9 years, he had otherwise been well, though he was said to be "clumsy" and to have been slow at running, "like his father." No other information concerning his maternal family history of hereditary neuropathy has emerged.

On examination, the patient does not have any mental status or other findings that might be related to the MRI lesion, but he now has some signs of distal muscle wasting of intrinsic hand muscles, is diffusely hyporeflexic, and has grade 4+ weakness in his grip and wrist extension. Sensory testing indicates a mild large fiber (proprioceptive) deficit in distal limbs, and gait testing shows that he has more difficulty walking on his heels than his toes (weak ankle dorsiflexion).

The MRI lesion might suggest some kind of incidental finding, unrelated to the patient's neuropathy—an isolated demyelinative lesion? Atypical (asymmetrical) adrenoleukodystrophy? But the absence of a clinical syndrome weighs against those possibilities. The MRI difference is most likely evidence that he has the X-linked type of CMT disease, since it is well established that this subtype, being a multiple-level (central plus peripheral) disorder of the nervous system, can be associated with fluctuating, monophasic white matter lesions. At this point, the patient not only is clearly symptomatic from an apparent hereditary neuropathy but also has a superimposed brain lesion that itself demands diagnostic clarification. It is appropriate to proceed with focused neurogenetic testing for mutations in connexin 32, the gene underlying most cases of X-linked CMT disease.

The patient is found to have a previously recognized mutation in the connexin 32 gene. CMT-X typically causes a mixed axonal/demyelinative neuropathy with a course similar to the more common dominantly inherited types of CMT (PMP22, which is demyelinative; axonal types). A 10-year prognosis could estimate that he will continue with the moderate functional limitations (e.g., in terms of competitiveness in sports, liability to injury due to proprioceptive loss) that the patient and his family have already come to know. Next steps include referral for genetic counseling, referral for physical therapy, and arrangements for follow-up in a multidisciplinary neuromuscular clinic.

Unlike many X-linked disorders, CMT-X commonly manifests in female "carriers" of the mutation. The discussion turns to whether your patient's 6-year-old sister should be tested. While there could be different reasonable responses to this question, a common response could emphasize stepping back from presymptomatic genetic testing in a child, a principle guiding the diagnostic decision making at the initial visit in this case. The increasing use of "next-generation" diagnostic sequencing technologies will undoubtedly have an impact on the ethics and diagnostic practices for neurogenetic diseases.

> **KEY POINTS TO REMEMBER**
> - Hereditary neuropathy may follow several different inheritance patterns; demyelinative types are more common than axonopathies..
> - Genetic testing can help confirm the diagnosis and anticipate manifestations and course of the condition..
> - X-linked CMT may present with white matter lesions of the brain on MRI.

Further Reading

Abrams CK, Freidin M. GJB1-associated X-linked Charcot-Marie-Tooth disease, a disorder affecting the central and peripheral nervous systems. *Cell Tissue Res* 2015;360:659–73.

El-Abassi R, England JD, Carter GT. Charcot-Marie-Tooth disease: an overview of genotypes, phenotypes, and clinical management strategies. *Phys Med Rehab* 2014;6:342–55.

Meriem Tazir M, Hamadouche T, Nouioua S, Mathis S, Vallat J. Hereditary motor and sensory neuropathies or Charcot–Marie–Tooth diseases: An update. *J Neurol Sci* 2014;347:14–22.

# 12  Of Cramped Limbs and a Rough Start

You are called to the neonatal intensive care unit (NICU) to see a 2-day-old boy with arthrogryposis. You learn that the child was the product of a 34-week pregnancy complicated by polyhydramnios and reduced fetal movements. The labor was prolonged and forceps delivery was eventually required. The infant had respiratory distress at birth and required a few minutes of ventilatory assistance with an Ambu bag in the delivery room. The neonatologists are concerned about a decreased activity level and poor feeding.

When you arrive in the NICU you find a child who is at the 3rd percentile for weight, height, and head circumference. The child appears dysmorphic, with a V-shaped mouth (upper lip forms an inverted V) and a paucity of facial expression (facial diplegia). The child is hypotonic, has absent reflexes, and has joint contractures at the elbow, knees, and ankles (arthrogryposis multiplex congenita). The child has a poor suck. Despite these findings, the child looks remarkably alert. He follows well and responds to noxious stimuli with a cry, albeit a weak one.

**What do you do now?**

## CONGENITAL MYOTONIC DYSTROPHY

Arthrogryposis multiplex congenita has a broad differential diagnosis, featuring an array of disorders primarily affecting the brain, the peripheral nervous system, or both. This child's hypotonia appears most likely to stem from a problem with the peripheral nervous system (anterior horn cell, nerve, muscle, neuromuscular junction), considering the constellation of findings: arreflexia, tent-like mouth, and alert mental status. The differential diagnosis would include

- A congenital neuropathy such as hypomyelinating neuropathy
- Spinal muscular atrophy
- One of the congenital muscular dystrophies
- Metabolic myopathies such as acid maltase deficiency
- Maternal transmission of acetylcholine receptor antibody (congenital autoimmune myasthenia)
- One of the congenital myopathies (central core disease, congenital fiber-type disproportion myopathy, minicore disease, myotubular myopathy, nemaline rod myopathy)

Before doing an extensive evaluation on the child, the mother should be examined for any possible weakness. When you examine the mother, you note some frontal bossing and mild facial diplegia (Fig. 12–1). When queried, the mother describes difficulty opening jars and turning doorknobs. When asked to squeeze your fingers and then let go, the mother has difficulty relaxing her grip. When her thenar eminence is struck with a hammer, myotonia is induced (Fig. 12–2).

These findings make it overwhelmingly likely that the mother has myotonic dystrophy and the child has congenital myotonic dystrophy. The diagnosis can be confirmed by genetic analysis. Myotonic dystrophy is a multisystem disorder transmitted by autosomal dominant inheritance. An expanded CTG repeat in the *DMPK* gene (chromosome 19q13.2–13.3) causes this dominant disorder, for which the severity of the phenotype is roughly proportional to the number of CTG repeats. The CTG mutation is itself unstable, such that the number of repeats may change from generation to generation. Amplified CTG repeat number are more often passed from mother to child than from father to child; this is why the mother is usually the affected parent when the newborn has the disorder.

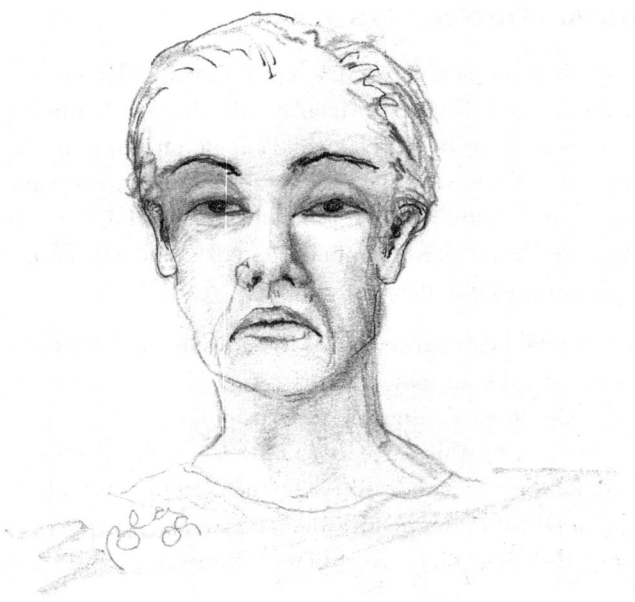

**FIGURE 12-1** Frontal bossing and high hairline in mother with myotonic dystrophy.

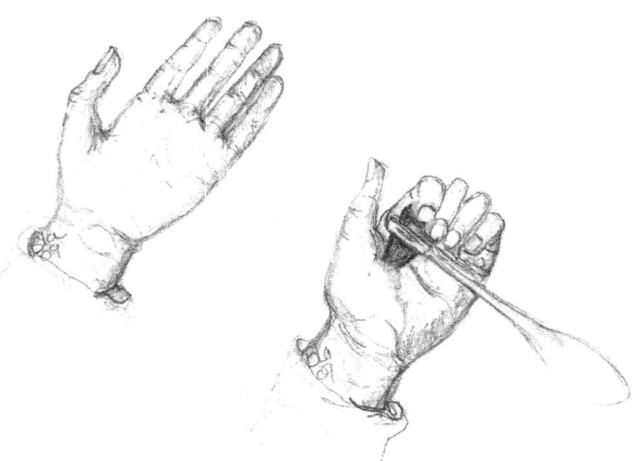

**FIGURE 12-2** When the thenar eminence is struck with a reflex hammer, myotonia occurs and the thumb gets "stuck" in the palm.

Myotonic dystrophy type 1 (DM1) is distinguished from the more variable type 2 (DM2), which features cardiac problems less often and is due to a mutation in a different gene. These are both multisystem disorders that are associated with cognitive impairment with brain MRI abnormalities, cardiac conduction abnormalities, a tendency to diabetes, and, later in life, cataracts. The overall average survival in DM1 is near 54 years of age, although patients with neonatal onset have a substantially shorter life expectancy.

While there is no direct therapy for the condition, physical therapy and orthopedic intervention can be very helpful.

> **KEY POINTS TO REMEMBER**
> - Infants born to mothers with myotonic dystrophy are at risk for significant problems.
> - Arthrogryposis, hypotonia, facial diplegia, and hyporeflexia are often presenting features, although other disorders may overlap this presentation.
> - Examining the mother usually will establish the diagnosis.
> - DNA testing is fairly reliable.

Further Reading

Johnston HM. The floppy weak infant revisited. *Brain Dev* 2003;25:155–8.

Jones HR, Jr., Darras BT. Acute care pediatric electromyography. *Muscle Nerve* 2000;Suppl 9:S53–62.

Meola G, Cardani R. Myotonic dystrophies: an update on clinical aspects, genetic, pathology, and molecular pathomechanisms. *Biochim Biophys Acta* 2015;1852:594–606.

Minnerop M, Weber B, Schoene-Bake J-C, et al. The brain in myotonic dystrophy 1 and 2: evidence for a predominant white matter disease. *Brain* 2011;134(12):3527–43. doi:10.1093/brain/awr299.

Prasad AN, Prasad C. The floppy infant: contribution of genetic and metabolic disorders. *Brain Dev* 2003;25:457–76.

Turner C, Hilton-Jones D. Myotonic dystrophy: diagnosis, management and new therapies. *Curr Opin Neurol* 2014;27:599–60.

# 13 The Case of the Changing Gait

A 6-year-old girl is referred for problems with walking. The mother stated that the child never walked or ran normally. She tells you that the girl began walking at 18 months but was always clumsy and frequently fell, particularly when she was tired at the end of the day. The mother was initially told by her primary care physician that her daughter may have a mild form of cerebral palsy.

Over the past 2 years her condition has worsened. The mother notes that when the child walks, she intermittently switches from normal heel to toe walking when tired. In addition, she turns both feet inward when walking. Over the past several months she has had numerous bruises from falling. The mother became increasingly worried when the girl had some unusual stiffening of her right arm when she was walking or running. When the mother discusses her concerns with her pediatrician, he tells her that this cannot be cerebral palsy and sends the child to you for evaluation. You learn that the child was born after a normal pregnancy, labor, and delivery. The mother feels her daughter is bright, and she is doing well in the first grade. The child has a 1-year-old brother who is developing normally. A family history of neurological disorders could not be elicited. The mother emphasizes to you that her daughter walks much better in the morning than in the afternoon.

On the morning of the examination you find a delightful, precocious girl who seems quite bright. Cranial nerves II–XII are normal. There is no nystagmus. Finger-to-nose is done accurately and without tremor. Her strength is normal. Her reflexes are normal and her plantar response to stimulation was flexor. When she walks she had some mild in-turning of the right foot. Her gait was awkward and rather stiff. The mother tells you that on the morning you examine the child she is doing well and that later in the day she expects that her walking will become much worse.

### What do you do now?

## DOPAMINE-RESPONSIVE DYSTONIA

The pediatrician is correct: the progressive course of the disorder as described by the mother makes it very unlikely that this child has cerebral palsy, which, though it can pose new, sometimes increasing challenges to the developing child, is by definition a static disorder. The variation in severity of the gait disturbance over the course of the day described by the mother is an intriguing observation, so you ask the parent to record some of her child's walking on her cellphone camera, and schedule the patient to come to your office in the late afternoon. Since there is a history that the gait abnormality is worse when she has exercised or is tired, you ask the mother to keep her very active before the appointment.

Three days later you see the patient, and the findings have changed considerably from the prior visit. When the child walks into your room you immediately notice that there has been a dramatic deterioration in gait. The child struggles to walk into the room. The right foot is turned inward to such a degree that the child is walking on the side of her foot and both legs are stiff. You also note that there is a decreased arm swing—both arms are rigidly extended, with the hands pronated. The hypertonus is of such a degree that it is difficult to bend the arms or legs. The child, while not in pain, clearly appears distressed by the muscle stiffness.

You recognize that you are dealing with dystonia, which as a descriptive, heterogeneous diagnosis is characterized by abnormal tonicity of muscle, with prolonged, repetitive muscle contractions, often involving simultaneous contractions of both agonists and antagonists, leading to twisting of the extremities.

The diverse causes of dystonia include structural and metabolic abnormalities, so you order an MRI of the head and blood studies (Table 13.1). However, the diurnal variation supports a strong suspicion that the child has dopamine-responsive dystonia, so you start the child on levodopa/carbidopa 25/100 mg bid while you are waiting for the results to return. A week later, the mother brings the child back and she is ecstatic. Since starting the levodopa/carbidopa the child is walking much better and for most of the day can run without a limp. The mother feels the drug has resulted in a miracle.

This patient likely has dopamine- or dopa-responsive dystonia, also known as hereditary progressive dystonia with diurnal variation, or Segawa

TABLE 13.1  **Differential Diagnosis of Episodic Dystonia in Children**

| Diagnosis | Comments |
| --- | --- |
| Paroxysmal kinesogenic choreoathetosis | Characterized by episodes of chorea, athetosis, or dystonia, triggered by sudden movements or startle. Episodes may be preceded by an aura and generally last seconds to minutes, although they do not involve loss of consciousness. The frequency of attacks varies considerably, from multiple times in a day to as few as once a month. |
| Paroxysmal nonkinesogenic choreoathetosis | Attacks of dystonia, chorea, athetosis, and ballismus that occur spontaneously. The condition manifests as attacks lasting from a few minutes to several hours. Episodes happen only when the individual is awake, and he or she remains conscious throughout the attack. Episodes can occur multiple times per day or there may be weeks or months between attacks. |
| Exercise-induced dystonia | A clinical condition characterized by dystonic postures in parts of the body, most commonly affecting the lower limbs, after prolonged exercise, lasting 5–30 minutes and disappearing (in most cases) within minutes of cessation of the physical activity. |
| Alternating hemiplegia | A condition where children have alternating periods of hemiparesis lasting from seconds to hours. Dystonia may be the principal manifestation during attacks. |
| Paroxysmal torticollis of infancy | A self-limited and benign entity characterized by recurrent episodes of head tilt, sometimes accompanied by vomiting, pallor, agitation, and ataxia, which subside spontaneously within a few hours or days and entirely disappear within months or years. |
| Ataxia-telangiectasia | Associated immunodeficiency (low IgG subclasses), elevated alpha fetoprotein, recessive inheritance. |

disease. An inherited dystonia typically presenting in the first decade of life, dopa-responsive dystonia is characterized by diurnal fluctuations, exquisite responsiveness to levodopa, and mild parkinsonian features. Adults with the disorder may be prone to impulsiveness, and cognitive impairment may be present in approximately 50% of cases.

This disorder is characterized by striatal dopamine deficiency with preservation of nigrostriatal terminals and is most frequently due to a dominantly inherited mutation of the GTP cyclohydrolase I (GCH) gene on chromosome 14q 22.1–22.2. However, about 40% of patients with dopamine-responsive dystonia have no identifiable mutation of the GCH gene. Other inherited conditions such as mutations in the tyrosine hydroxylase gene, aromatic L-amino acid decarboxylase and other defects of dopamine synthesis, tyrosine hydroxylase, sepiapterin reductase, or tetrahydrobiopterin metabolism can lead to dopamine-responsive dystonia.

There is considerable variation in the age of onset of the disorder as well as the severity of the condition. The early signs, as in this child, typically involve a disorder of gait that fluctuates in intensity during the course of the day. Marked gait difficulties can occur, and it is not uncommon for the child to be mistakenly diagnosed with cerebral palsy of the spastic diplegia type. Typically, the onset is in the first decade of life.

Dopamine production increases through the night with each cycle of rapid eye movement sleep. The activity at the nigrostriatal terminals peaks in the early morning and decreases during the day. Dopamine activity in the nigrostriatal terminals is reduced in patients with dopamine-responsive dystonia. This dopamine activity declines further during the day, leading to exacerbation of symptoms toward evening. It also decreases with increasing age, and thus the dystonia progressively worsens with age in many patients.

### KEY POINTS TO REMEMBER

- Cerebral palsy is a static disorder. If there is neurological deterioration, you are not dealing with cerebral palsy.
- Fluctuation of the severity of the dystonia during the course of day is characteristic of dopamine-responsive dystonia, with the symptoms worsening toward the end of the day.

- If untreated the condition is progressive, but if diagnosed and treated early, patients do quite well.
- Because the disorder in inherited it is very important for the clinician to take a detailed family history in order to identify other affected family members.

Further Reading

Albanese A, Bhatia K, Bressman SB, et al. Phenomenology and classification of dystonia: A consensus update. *Movement Disord* 2013;28:863–73.

Furukawa Y. Update on dopa-responsive dystonia: locus heterogeneity and biochemical features. *Adv Neurol* 2004;94:127–38.

Jan MM. Misdiagnoses in children with dopa-responsive dystonia. *Pediatr Neurol* 2004;31:298–303.

Jankovic J. Treatment of dystonia. *Lancet Neurol* 2006;5:864–72.

Lopez-Laso E, Sanchez-Raya A, Moriana JA, et al. Neuropsychiatric symptoms and intelligence quotient in autosomal dominant Segawa disease. *J Neurol* 2011;258:2155–62.

Segawa M, Hosaka A, Miyagawa F, et al. Hereditary progressive dystonia with marked diurnal fluctuation. *Adv Neurol* 1976;14:215–33.

Wijemanne S, Jankovic J. Dopa-responsive dystonia-clinical and genetic heterogeneity. *Nature Rev Neurol* 2015;11:414–24.

## 14 The Boy Who Couldn't Keep Up

You are called by a pediatrician to discuss a 5-year-old boy whose parents feel he may have cerebral palsy. The pediatrician tells you he has followed the child since birth. Although the boy was somewhat late in walking (16 months), the pediatrician felt this was a normal variant. However, recently the parents raised concern about his inability to keep up with his 3-year-old sister and they observe that he often walks up on his toes and seems to "waddle." The pediatrician is not concerned but wishes to run the case by you.

**What do you do now?**

## DUCHENNE MUSCULAR DYSTROPHY

Even though parents are often apologetic about comparing their children's developmental skills, such comparisons can sometimes provide clues to an important neurological problem. In this patient it would be important to see the family and examine the child. You arrange for an appointment in 3 weeks.

When you see the child you learn that not only did your patient walk later than his sister, who was walking at 9 months, but his speech also came later, and he has been enrolled in speech therapy for a mild expressive speech delay. The parents feel that compared to his sister he is quite clumsy. On examination, you find that the child is alert and interactive, wanting to explore the latex gloves and diagnostic instruments. Other than some moderate dysarthria (speech is about 80% intelligible), cranial nerve examination is normal. On muscle testing you find some probable mild weakness of the deltoids of the upper extremities (it is unclear if he is mounting a full effort) and more significant weakness of the proximal muscles of the lower extremities. Toe-walking and enlargement of the gastrocnemius muscles are observed. Tendon reflexes are difficult to elicit. When you ask the child to sit on the floor and then stand, he keeps his hands on the floor as he places his feet under him, and seems a little slow to come upright, although he doesn't show a full Gower sign (i.e., using his hands and arms to push up to a standing position; Fig. 14–1).

This child likely has Duchenne muscular dystrophy, a dystrophinopathy. As in this child, the early symptoms are insidious and often dismissed by pediatricians and parents. Children with Duchenne muscular dystrophy may present with developmental delay, particularly in speech. Concerns regarding motor development may arise first when it is apparent that the child's running is slower than that of his or her peers or when the child seems to fatigue easily or shows increasing toe-walking. In this context, toe-walking reflects the selectivity of the myopathy, as it involves foot dorsiflexors (anterior tibialis) more than plantar flexors. The majority of children maintain their ability to walk and climb stairs until 8 years of age. Eventually boys with Duchenne muscular dystrophy develop progressive loss of gait (typically by age 10), with compromise of respiratory muscles

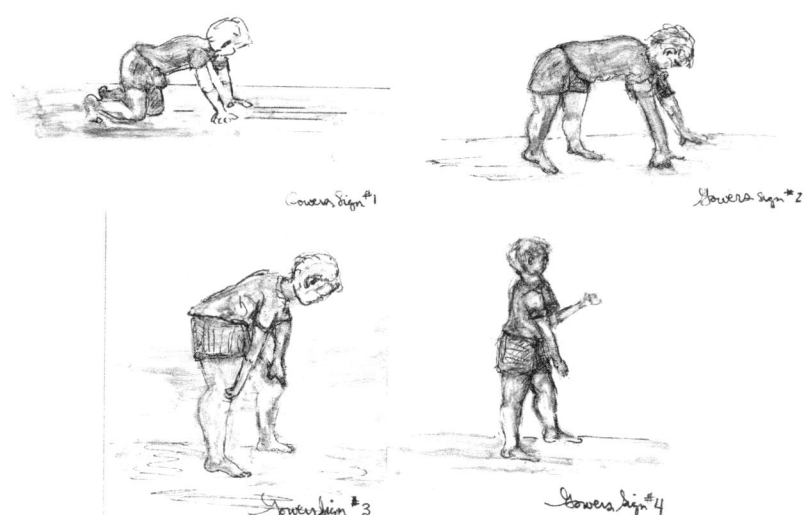

**FIGURE 14–1** Gower sign. Because of proximal leg weakness, the child uses his hands and arms to climb up his legs to get to a standing position.

(restrictive lung disease), dilated cardiomyopathy, loss of tendon reflexes, and severe proximal weakness of both the upper and lower extremities.

Cerebral palsy can present with gait disturbances, but it represents a variety of static, brain-based disorders of motor control, so that hyperreflexia, spasticity, and dystonia (with rarer cases featuring ataxia, choreoathetosis, or hypotonia) are the typical physical findings. While there can be some phenotypic overlap, Becker muscular dystrophy, also due to a mutation in the dystrophin gene, can be differentiated from Duchenne muscular dystrophy by its later age of onset (older than 5 years). Boys with Becker dystrophy may still show unassisted ambulation after age 15 and may survive into adult life. Muscle biopsy shows more dystrophin in children with Becker muscular dystrophy than those with Duchenne muscular dystrophy. Table 14.1 lists the major muscular dystrophies of childhood.

Duchenne muscular dystrophy is a genetic disorder due to a genetic defect at the Xp21 site. The dystrophin mutation leads to instability of the sarcolemmal membrane due to reduced muscle content of the structural, membrane-linked protein dystrophin. In both Becker and Duchenne dystrophy, loss of sarcolemma membrane integrity causes markedly elevation

TABLE 14.1 **Muscular Dystrophies of Childhood**

| Type | Comment |
|---|---|
| *Dystrophin-related disorders* | |
| Duchenne/Becker muscular dystrophy | Becker muscular dystrophy is an allelic, milder form of Duchenne muscular dystrophy. |
| Severe childhood autosomal recessive muscular dystrophy | Phenotypically identical to Duchenne muscular dystrophy but with normal dystrophin content in muscle. Occurs in both sexes. |
| *Non–dystrophin-related disorders* | |
| Emery-Dreifuss muscular dystrophy | X-linked condition with contractures, weakness, cardiomyopathy |
| Facioscapulohumeral dystrophy | Facial diplegia, progressive proximal weakness, first affecting the shoulders and then the pelvis, often asymmetrical |
| Limb-girdle muscular dystrophy | X-linked disorder with progressive proximal muscle weakness |
| *Congenital muscular dystrophy* | |
| Merosin-deficient muscular dystrophy | Striking, T2 bright lesions on head MRI; moderate CK elevation |
| Fukuyama congenital muscular dystrophy | Early-life onset of proximal weakness, hypotonia, absent reflexes, seizures, developmental delay |
| Walker-Warburg syndrome | Severe lissencephaly, epilepsy, intellectual impairment, eye abnormalities such as corneal clouding, cataracts, retinal detachment, hypotonia, and weakness |
| Muscle-eye-brain (Santavuori) syndrome | Cortical dysplasia, epilepsy, intellectual impairment, complex eye abnormalities, weakness, contractures, and hypotonia |

of creatine kinase (CK) levels (10 or more times normal). Following such a "screening" laboratory result, the diagnosis of Duchenne muscular dystrophy can readily be confirmed by genetic analysis. While a muscle biopsy, and follow-on immunohistochemical testing for tissue dystrophin, can also provide the diagnosis, such testing is often obviated by a definitive dystrophin mutation from blood DNA testing.

While Duchenne muscular dystrophy is not curable, it is treatable. Daily prednisone treatment (0.75 mg/kg/day), if well tolerated (watch for weight gain) in conjunction with physical therapy can increase the duration of ambulation by about 1 year.

> **KEY POINTS TO REMEMBER**
> - There is mild early motor delay; onset is insidious.
> - Children may present with speech delay; observe the gait carefully.
> - This is a multisystem disorder that features cardiac involvement and intellectual impairment.
> - Becker muscular dystrophy has a later onset and a milder course.
> - Waddling gait, enlarged calf muscles, and the Gower sign are keys to the diagnosis.
> - Mutational analysis can confirm the diagnosis and can inform genetic counseling.

Further Reading

Birnkrant DJ. The American College of Chest Physicians Consensus Statement on the Respiratory and Related Management of Patients With Duchenne Muscular Dystrophy Undergoing Anesthesia or Sedation. *Pediatrics* 2009;123:S242–4.

Katharine Bushby K et al. Diagnosis and management of Duchenne muscular dystrophy, part 1: diagnosis, and pharmacological and psychosocial management. Lancet Neurol 2010; 9: 77–93

Emery AE. Muscular dystrophy into the new millennium. *Neuromuscul Disord* 2002;12:343–9.

Manzur AY, Kinali M, Muntoni F. Update on the management of Duchenne muscular dystrophy. *Arch Dis Child* 2008;93:986–90.

Manzur AY, Muntoni F. Diagnosis and new treatments in muscular dystrophies. *J Neurol Neurosurg Psychiatry* 2009;80:706–14.

Moxley RT, Ashwal S, Pandya S, et al. Practice Parameter: Corticosteroid treatment of Duchenne dystrophy—Report of the Quality Standards Subcommittee of the American Academy of Neurology and the Practice Committee of the Child Neurology Society. *Neurology* 2005;64:13–20.

Prior TW, Bridgeman SJ. Experience and strategy for the molecular testing of Duchenne muscular dystrophy. *J Mol Diagn* 2005;7:317–26.

# 15 Beyond Autism: A Genetic Resolution

You are called by a local pediatrician who wishes you to see a 6-year-old boy with autism who had a generalized tonic-clonic seizure. You learn from the pediatrician that the child was born after a full-term pregnancy to a G3P2 → 3 mom who had no difficulties with the spontaneous vaginal delivery. The child weighed 3,200 grams and had good Apgar scores. The mother was concerned about his development beginning with the first year of life. Compared to his 8-year-old brother and 9-year-old sister, he was never quite "right," even during the first year of life, when he rarely smiled and was delayed in rolling over, sitting, and walking.

When you see the child, the parents tell you that he was given a diagnosis of autism a year ago because of a combination of language delay, poor social interactions, and some self-stimulatory behavior, including hand biting. As you take the history you observe that the boy is quite hyperactive and disruptive to the point where the grandmother has to take the child out of the examining room. Once the child leaves the mother tells you he will be held back in kindergarten for another year. He is substantially delayed. He does not know his colors, can count only to six, and does not know his birthday, address, or phone number. The mother says he has a short temper and is argumentative and aggressive with members of the family.

Two weeks prior to your office visit the boy was found in the early morning having a generalized tonic-clonic seizure. The child's eyes were opened, with rhythmic jerking of the arms and legs. The parents describe perioral cyanosis and incontinence. The seizure lasted approximately 2 minutes. When seen in the local emergency room he had a glucose level, electrolytes, CBC, and MRI, all of which were normal. He was started on phenytoin.

When you bring the child back into the room he physically opposes the examination and makes little if any eye contact with you. He does not follow commands and shows little interest in you, preferring to explore the room. His head circumference is normal, although he has a prominent forehead and jaw. The neurological examination is otherwise normal, although visualizing the fundi is not possible.

### What do you do now?

## FRAGILE X SYNDROME

This child likely has fragile X syndrome, a disorder with a mutation on the X chromosome that was originally identified in males, although females may have a phenotype with a milder degree of intellectual impairment. Clues to the diagnosis are the developmental delay in a boy, his unusual face, and his autistic, hyperactive behaviors. In this child the first step is to order genetic testing, a trinucleotide repeat sequence mutation in the fragile X gene, *FMR-1*. Considering the first unprovoked seizure, an EEG could be considered, although the likelihood of a consequential finding must be weighed against the stress, for patient and technicians alike, of technically setting up the EEG.

Boys with fragile X syndrome have a wide range of intellectual impairment, with IQ ranging from 20 to 80. In addition, many have features of autistic spectrum disorder, consisting of abnormalities in social interaction and communication and repetitive behaviors or interests. Attention-deficit/hyperactivity disorder and conduct disorders are also common in the condition. Macro-orchidism can be an important clue to the diagnosis for the syndrome, but this may not be evident until after puberty. Not all boys have the originally described craniofacial dysmorphism, so that testing may be considered in any boy with otherwise unexplained intellectual impairment.

Although progress in understanding the pathobiology of this condition increasingly holds the promise of targeted therapy, and numerous drug trials are under way based on evidence of disrupted glutamatergic and GABA-ergic signaling. Meanwhile, medical care for an individual with fragile X syndrome focuses on treating common problems such as anxiety, gastroesophageal reflux, sleep disturbance, otitis, and autism (seen in 40% to 60%). Epilepsy occurs in approximately 25% of the boys and is usually not difficult to control. However, phenytoin would not be an ideal drug due to its association with behavioral (hyperactivity, irritability) and disfiguring (lymphoidal hypertrophy, acromegalic facial features) side effects. The EEG findings in this condition vary; some children have centrotemporal spikes.

Fragile X syndrome is caused by an expansion of a CGG repeat in the *FMR1* gene resulting in the absence of the *FMR1* mRNA and protein.

The fragile X DNA assay has greatly improved both the sensitivity and the specificity of fragile X diagnosis. Since chromosome analysis may be falsely negative, DNA testing is important. The *FMR1* protein is proposed to act as a regulator of mRNA transport and of translation of target mRNAs at the synapse. Both males and females can be affected: about 25% of females with the mutation have an IQ of less than 70, and most of the others have borderline or low-normal IQ.

> **KEY POINTS TO REMEMBER**
> - Fragile X is the most common single-gene cause of intellectual impairment in males (nonspecific, familial intellectual impairment is more common).
> - Epilepsy occurs in approximately 20% to 25% of the children.
> - A normal karyotype analysis does not rule out fragile X syndrome; DNA testing is required.
> - Consider testing females with intellectual impairment if the inheritance pattern fits with an X-linked disorder.

Further Reading

Cornish K, Turk J, Hagerman R. The fragile X continuum: new advances and perspectives. *J Intellect Disabil Res* 2008;52:469–82.

Hagerman RJ. Translating molecular advances in fragile X syndrome into therapy: a review. *J Clin Psychiatry* 2014;75(4):e294–e307.

Hagerman RJ, Berry-Kravis E, Kaufmann WE, et al. Advances in the treatment of fragile X syndrome. *Pediatrics* 2009;123:378–90.

Hagerman RJ, Ono MY, Hagerman PJ. Recent advances in fragile X: a model for autism and neurodegeneration. *Curr Opin Psychiatry* 2005;18:490–6.

Kidd SA, Lachiewicz A, Barbouth D, et al. Fragile X syndrome: a review of associated medical problems. *Pediatrics* 2014;134:995–1005.

Rousseau F. The fragile X syndrome: implications of molecular genetics for the clinical syndrome. *Eur J Clin Invest* 1994;24:1–10.

# 16 Learning Difficulty: Diagnosis Beyond the Neurological Examination

A pediatrician refers an 8-year-old girl to you because of concerns about development. The child was the product of a normal labor and uneventful vaginal delivery to a 25-year-old, healthy G1P1 mother. The child weighed 3,400 grams (50th percentile), had a head circumference of 35 cm (50th percentile), and had Apgar scores of 9/10. You learn from the parents that the girl reached all motor developmental milestones on time but did not use understandable words until age 2, and she did not use phrases until age 3 (Table 16.1).

The girl was deemed to be slow in school and while in second grade had an aide and an individual education plan (IEP). She underwent psychological testing in the first grade, and the parents were told she was delayed by about a year, with her greatest difficulty in expressive and receptive speech. The parents say she is uncoordinated and does not do well in team sports such as soccer. She prefers playing with younger children. Her general health has been excellent, without any hospitalization or head trauma. The results of her earlier lead and hearing screenings were satisfactory. Both parents completed college and there is no family history of intellectual impairment or learning deficits.

When you observe the girl, you find that she is slow in responding and has a limited fund of knowledge for her age. For example, she cannot tell time, and is unaware of the year she was born or the current date or day of the week. She has frequent restless, fidgety movements, and has difficulty staying on task. She attempts to read a paragraph from a first-grade book but is very slow and makes many errors. She cannot tell you if she is right- or left-handed.

On examination you find that while her weight and height are at the 40th percentile, she has a large head (56 cm, greater than the 95th percentile). Cranial nerve examination is normal. She demonstrates dysdiadochokinesia with rapid alternating movements and has difficulty jumping on each foot. Muscle stretch reflexes, muscle strength testing, and sensory examination are normal. She shows overflow movements in her upper extremities when toe or heel walking (fingers pointing downward or upward, respectively), and she has trouble catching a bounced ball.

### What do you do now?

TABLE 16.1  Important Developmental Milestones During First 3 Years of Life

| 1 Month | 3 Months | 6 Months | 12 Months | 24 Months | 36 Months |
|---|---|---|---|---|---|
| Moves head from side to side while lying on stomach | Raises head and chest when lying on stomach | Reaches for object and brings to mouth | Drinks from a cup with help | Take off clothes | Drinks from a straw |
| Keeps hands in tight fists | Supports upper body with arms when lying on stomach | Good head control when in the sitting position | Feeds self finger foods | Scribbles with crayons | Feeds self with a spoon |
| Strong reflex movements | Pushes down on legs when feet are placed on a firm surface | Explores by mouthing and banging objects | Develops pincer grasp | Walks and runs without help | Washes hands |
| Focuses 8–12 inches away | Brings hand to mouth | Sits with minimal support | Points | Identifies an object in a picture book | Partially dresses self |
| Recognizes some sounds | Grasps and shakes hand toys | Rolls over | Puts small blocks in and takes them out of a container | Looks and searches for objects that are out of sight | Builds a tower of 3 or 4 blocks |
| | Follows moving objects | Knows familiar faces | Bangs blocks | Follows one-step directions | Throws ball |
| | Recognizes familiar objects and people at a distance | Laughs and squeals with delight | Sits well without support | Has expressive vocabulary of 8–10 words | Stoops and recovers |
| | Begins to babble | Smiles at self in a mirror | Crawls on hands and knees | Looks at a person who is talking to him/her | Walks up steps |
| | Turns head toward direction of sound | | Pulls to stand | Uses "hi," "bye," and "please," with reminders | Walks backward |
| | Begins to develop a social smile | | Walks with one hand held | Recognizes self in the mirror or in pictures | Points to 5 or 6 body parts |
| | | | Copies sounds | | Has a vocabulary of several hundred words |
| | | | Say first word | | Uses 2- to 3-word sentences |
| | | | Shows separation anxiety from parent | | Refers to self by name and uses "me" and "mine" |
| | | | Understand simple commands | | Verbalizes desires ("I want juice") |

## NEUROFIBROMATOSIS

There are numerous causes for developmental delay, and many clinicians struggle in terms of how extensively a child should be evaluated. In this case you learn that while the child has cognitive problems, there has been no developmental regression. Knowing you are dealing with a static problem is helpful in eliminating an evaluation for a degenerative problem and directs your evaluation toward static conditions.

Before embarking on a costly evaluation, you should consider possible clues from the case. The best predictor of a child's intelligence is the intelligence of the mother. Since both parents are cognitively normal, there clearly is a process here that goes beyond familial traits. The observation that the child has macrocephaly should lead you to measure both of the parents' head size, since macrocephaly may run in families and be of no clinical significance. Both of her parents have normal head circumferences.

An essential part of every examination of a child with a learning disability is an examination of the skin. When you have the child disrobe you find that she has six café-au-lait spots greater than 5 mm in diameter and axillary freckling (Fig. 16–1).

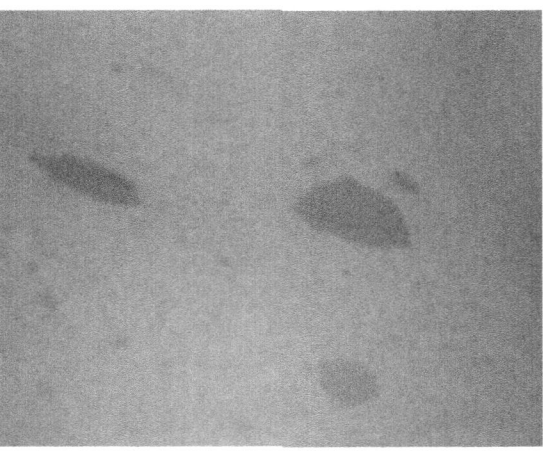

**FIGURE 16-1** Café-au-lait spots in a child with neurofibromatosis.

Based on these simple findings on the physical examination—intertriginous freckling is vanishingly rare outside of neurocutaneous disease—this child has type 1 neurofibromatosis (NF1). NF1 is a neurocutaneous syndrome characterized by peripheral (neurofibromas, schwannomas) or central (gliomatous) tumors. The abnormal gene for NF1 is located on chromosome 17q and its abnormal protein product is neurofibromin. Over 100 mutations of the gene have been recognized, and almost 50% of these arise de novo. Despite the large number of mutations, commercial genetic screening for NF1 is available.

Box 16.1 lists the diagnostic features of NF. In this child the café-au-lait spots and freckling in the axillary region confirm the diagnosis of NF1. Macrocephaly is also common in the disorder. Although you did not note any Lisch nodules, it would be useful to arrange for yearly examination by an ophthalmologist, since in addition to Lisch nodules, which often appear later in life, these children are at risk for optic gliomas. Many of these, which tend to develop before age 6, remain asymptomatic, may regress spontaneously, and do not need treatment.

NF1 is a dominantly inherited genetic disorder of the nervous system that primarily affects the development and growth of neural crest–derived tissues. About half of all cases arise by spontaneous mutations. NF1 is associated with nerve tumors, which may be either nodular/pendular

---

BOX 16.1  **Diagnostic Criteria for Neurofibromatosis Type 1**

**Two or more are considered diagnostic:**

Six café-au-lait spots >5 mm in diameter in prepubertal individuals or >15 mm in postpubertal individuals
Two or more neurofibromas or one plexiform neurofibroma
Freckling in the axillary or inguinal region
Optic glioma
Two or more iris hamartomas (Lisch nodules)
A distinctive osseous lesion, such as sphenoid dysplasia or thinning of long bones
A first-degree relative with NF1

(neurofibromas) or plexiform. These tumors can be painful and disfiguring. Plexiform neurofibromas, typically arising in either the cervical or paraspinal areas, tend toward monotonous, indolent extension, rarely develop after adolescence, and can be particularly difficult to manage. Children with NF1 are also at risk for intraspinal neurofibromas, dural ectasia, and aqueductal stenosis. As in this girl, NF is associated with learning disabilities (approximately 50%).

In view of the large head and the risk for optic glioma, MRI screening of the head bears consideration, although routine MRI at initial NF1 diagnosis is not universally accepted. Although the MRI in this child proved to be normal, NF1 may be associated with areas of increased T2 signal, termed "unidentified bright objects," throughout the brain. The significance of such lesions is unclear.

NF1 is the more common type of the neurofibromatoses. NF2 does not feature pigmented cutaneous lesions. This condition is characterized by bilateral tumors on the eighth cranial nerve that cause pressure damage to neighboring nerves.

Treatment for NF1 is symptomatic. In most cases, symptoms of NF1 are mild and patients live normal lives, although with average life expectancy shortened by about 15 years, owing to increased liability to cancers, including neural tumors. Acquired vascular lesions can occur, and monitoring for hypertension is appropriate. Surgery can help some NF1 bone malformations and remove painful or disfiguring tumors; however, there is a chance that the tumors may grow back, and in greater numbers.

In the case presented here, having a diagnosis provides prognostic guidance for both the family and school. This condition features a high prevalence of attention-deficit/hyperactivity disorder (more than 50% by some estimates), so it will be worth evaluating for this pharmacologically amenable condition in children with NF1. With speech, occupational, and physical therapy combined with a patient-specific educational plan, the child can improve, although learning challenges will persist.

> **KEY POINTS TO REMEMBER**
>
> - Examing the skin for pigmented or hypopigmented macules (tuberous sclerosis complex) is important in the setting of intellectual impairment.
> - Children with NF1 are at risk for optic gliomas and brain tumors.
> - Screen children with NF1 carefully for attention-deficit disorder.

Further Reading

Acosta MT, Gioia GA, Silva AJ. Neurofibromatosis type 1: new insights into neurocognitive issues. *Curr Neurol Neurosci Rep* 2006;6:136–43.

Ferner RE, Huson SM, Thomas N, et al. Guidelines for the diagnosis and management of individuals with neurofibromatosis 1. *J Med Genet* 2007;44:81–8.

Gerber PA, Antal AS, Neumann NJ, et al. Neurofibromatosis. *Eur J Med Res* 2009;14:102–5.

Gilboa Y. Application of the International Classification of Functioning, Disability and Health in children with neurofibromatosis type 1: a review. *Developmental Medicine & Child Neurology* 2010;52:612–9

Jett K, Friedman JM. Clinical and genetic aspects of neurofibromatosis 1. *Genet Med* 2010;12(1):1–11.

Radtke HB, Sebold CD, Allison C, Haidle JL, Schneider G. Neurofibromatosis type 1 in genetic counseling practice: recommendations of the National Society of Genetic Counselors. *J Genet Couns* 2007;16:387–407.

# 17  A Sleepy Newborn

You get a call from the neonatal intensive care unit (NICU) to see a 3-day-old boy admitted because of possible clonic seizures. The child was a full-term infant born to a healthy 25-year-old mother. After a prolonged labor the child was delivered with vacuum extraction, with a birth weight of 3,000 g and Apgar scores of 3 at 1 minute, 7 at 5 minutes, and 8 at 10 minutes. The infant did well the first 24 hours after birth. However, on the second day of life, the nurses noted that the child awakened less frequently, and when awake was very irritable. That night, the evening-shift nurse noted intermittent rhythmic jerking of left, right, or both arms associated with facial twitching.

The neonatologists obtained a CBC, a C-reactive protein, and stat electrolytes and glucose level, all of which were normal. A spinal tap revealed a protein of 70 mg/dL, glucose of 50 mg/dL, and eight white blood cells, 60% of which were polymorphonuclear leukocytes. Blood and spinal fluid were sent for culture as the child was started on broad-spectrum antibiotics and loaded with phenobarbital intravenously (20 mg/kg). Within hours after receiving phenobarbital and antibiotics, the child became increasingly lethargic and would not feed. Periods of apnea and clonic movements of both arms and legs continued over the next 12 hours, as temperatures fluctuated from 36° to 38°C. On day 3, the neonatologists obtain a head ultrasound, which shows possible cerebral edema. They ask for your opinion, voicing concerns that the child is suffering from delayed symptoms of birth asphyxia.

When you examine the infant, you note lethargy—voice and tactile stimulation fail to awaken the hypotonic infant, whose eyes remain closed. The head circumference is normal. Pupils are pinpoint, making it difficult to do a funduscopic examination. With lids held open, the child had full range of movements with doll's-eye maneuver, and corneal reflexes are present. The child has a weak suck, and you cannot elicit a Moro, grasp, deep tendon reflexes, or plantar response.

**What do you do now?**

## ORNITHINE TRANSCARBAMYLASE DEFICIENCY

The overall picture is that of a late-onset (i.e., day 2) neonatal encephalopathy with seizures. As a syndrome with a variety of potential underlying pathologies, it is often useful to question the frequent assumption that neonatal encephalopathy is due to a hypoxic-ischemic stress. In this case, the history weighs against hypoxic-ischemic encephalopathy: the Apgar scores, while low at 1 minute, were well over the benchmark value of 5 at 5 minutes, and the child's behavior appears to have been normal during the first 24 hours. Laboratory values point away from sepsis or intracranial infection (cerebrospinal fluid formula is normal for a term infant) as the cause of encephalopathy. Despite the absence of reflexes, the lethargy, seizures, and temperature fluctuations suggest a disorder of the central rather than the peripheral nervous system. Progressive lethargy, with the onset of seizures after 24 hours, strongly suggest a metabolic encephalopathy (Table 17.1).

You recommend that the infant have an EEG and serum testing for organic acids, amino acids, lactate, liver function tests, and a blood ammonia.

The EEG, during which the infant remained asleep, without seizures, shows an excessively discontinuous EEG pattern with frequent multifocal spikes and sharp waves. Knowing that there can be a high "false positive" rate in the bedside diagnosis of neonatal seizures, the multifocal sharp activity increases your confidence that this patient should continue on phenobarbital, a standard practice in acute symptomatic neonatal seizures that still awaits evidence of impact on outcomes. The serum ammonia level was 650 µmol/L (normal 10 to 40 µmol/L). Serum amino acid quantification show elevated ornithine, glutamine, and alanine levels and relatively low citrulline levels. Urine organic acid studies show an elevated urinary orotic acid level. Lactic acid level is normal, and liver function tests show slight elevations.

The high blood ammonia level in the face of a normal serum glucose level and normal anion gap strongly suggests a urea cycle defect, which may be due to several different underlying enzymopathies. The elevated ornithine, glutamine, alanine, and orotic acid levels, coupled with a low citrulline level, indicate one of the more commonly recognized causes,

TABLE 17.1 **Common Causes of Neonatal Seizures as a Function of Age**

| Day 1 | Day 2 | Day 3 or Later |
|---|---|---|
| Hypoxia-ischemia | Postnatal infection | Cerebral dysgenesis |
| Trauma | Drug withdrawal | Cerebral venous thrombosis |
| Stroke | (from mother) | |
| Infection (bacterial or viral) | Cerebral dysgenesis | Inborn errors of metabolism |
| Intraventricular hemorrhage | Stroke | |
| Subarachnoid hemorrhage | Inborn errors of metabolism: | Intracerebral hemorrhage |
| Severe metabolic disturbance: | | |
| Non-ketotic hyperglycinemia | Urea cycle defects | Aminoacidopathies |
| Pyridoxine dependency | Glucose-transporter Defect | Organic acidurias: Methylmalonic aciduria |
| Sulfite oxidase | | Propionic acidemia |
| Hypoglycemia | | Maple syrup urine disease |
| Hypocalcemia | | |

ornithine transcarbamylase (OTC) deficiency (Fig. 17–1). Although relatively common among urea cycle disorders, OTC deficiency occurs in one out of every 14,000 to 80,000 births. This genetic disorder results in a mutated and ineffective form of the enzyme OTC, so that large levels of ammonia accumulate in the blood and brain. A definitive diagnosis of OTC deficiency is via determination of enzyme level from a liver biopsy, or by mutation analysis of the OTC gene.

As in this case, OTC deficiency typically becomes evident within days of birth. Infants with OTC deficiency typically develop lethargy, anorexia, irregular respiratory patterns, fluctuating body temperature, and seizures.

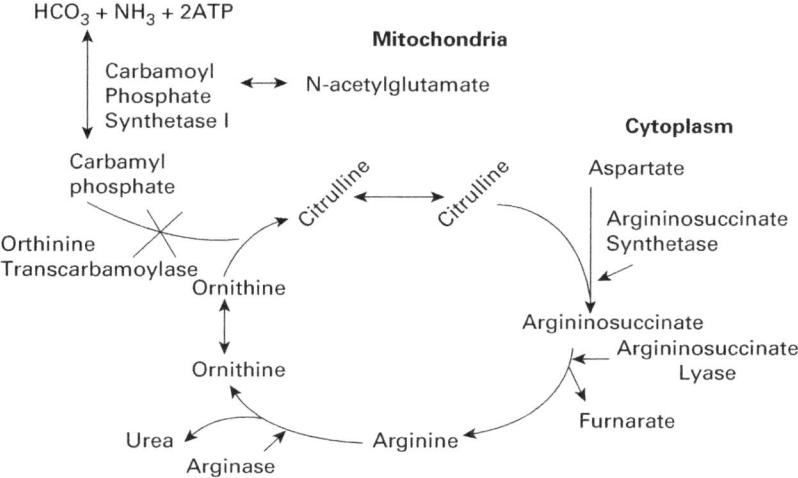

**FIGURE 17-1** Amino metabolism and the urea cycle. ARG, arginase; ASL, argininosuccinate lyase; ASS, argininosuccinate synthetase; CPSI, carbamoyl phosphate synthetase I; OTC, ornithine transcarbamylase. In this child OTC was deficient (marked by X), resulting in an increase of $NH_3$.

If untreated the infants typically go on to develop severe seizures, liver damage, and brain injury, including mental retardation, or death. In some affected individuals, signs and symptoms of OTC deficiency may be less severe and may not appear until later in life. With occasional exceptions featuring episodic hyperammonemia, studies showing cognitive impairment in so-called female carriers of this X-linked condition belie the term carrier, and some females may develop severe episodic hyperammonemia. The age of presentation in males depends on how the mutation affects gene function. Of particular relevance to the practice of pediatric neurology, otherwise asymptomatic males or females with OTC mutations may be particularly vulnerable to sodium valproate, among other metabolic stressors or illnesses.

With a serum blood ammonia this high, treatment must begin immediately, even before the specific diagnosis is made. Since the disease results in an inability to handle large amounts of a nitrogen load, the treatment includes strategies to remove excess ammonia, to decrease the intake of nitrogen (low-protein diet), to prevent excessive body protein breakdown during acute illnesses (hydration and nutrition), to reduce catabolism through the introduction of calories supplied by carbohydrates and fats rather than protein, and to scavenge nitrogen (sodium benzoate and sodium phenylacetate). Some centers have explored the use of therapeutic hypothermia in neonates with hyperammonemic encephalopathy due to urea cycle disorders. Liver transplant and supplemental amino acids (arginine, citrulline, valine, leucine, isoleucine) have also been used. Sadly, even with meticulous monitoring of blood ammonia, episodes of hyperammonemia may occur and lead to coma and death.

> **KEY POINTS TO REMEMBER**
> - OTC deficiency is one of several enzymopathies featuring hyperammonemia.
> - Severe forms of OTC present in the neonatal period, while mutations causing partial loss of enzyme function present later in life.
> - The infant with OTC may appear quite healthy at birth and then deteriorate over several days, with lethargy, anorexia, apnea, temperature fluctuations, seizures, and abnormal movements.
> - A high blood ammonia level in the face of a normal serum glucose level and normal anion gap strongly suggests a urea cycle defect.
> - Early recognition and treatment is critical to prevent severe brain damage and death.

Further Reading

Bergmann KR. Late-onset ornithine transcarbamylase deficiency: treatment and outcome of hyperammonemic crisis. *Pediatrics* 2013;133:e1072.

Burton BK. Inborn errors of metabolism: the clinical diagnosis in early infancy. *Pediatrics* 1987;79:359–69.

Burton BK. Inborn errors of metabolism in infancy: a guide to diagnosis. *Pediatrics* 1998;102:E69.

Cohn RM, Roth KS. Hyperammonemia, bane of the brain. *Clin Pediatr (Phila)* 2004;43:683–9.

Enns GM. Neurologic damage and neurocognitive dysfunction in urea cycle disorders. *Semin Pediatr Neurol* 2008;15:132–9.

Gordon N. Ornithine transcarbamylase deficiency: a urea cycle defect. *Eur J Paediatr Neurol* 2003;7:115-21.

Ogier de BH. Management and emergency treatments of neonates with a suspicion of inborn errors of metabolism. *Semin Neonatol* 2002;7:17-26.

Saudubray JM, Nassogne MC, de Lonlay P, Touati G. Clinical approach to inherited metabolic disorders in neonates: an overview. *Semin Neonatol* 2002;7:3-15.

Sprouse C. Investigating neurological deficits in carriers and affected patients with ornithine transcarbamylase deficiency. Mol Genet Metabol 2014;113:136-41.

# 18   A Loss of Connection

You are asked by concerned parents to evaluate their 2-year-old daughter. They state that the girl was fine until approximately age 12 months, when they noted that she had a decreased interest in her toys, reduced eye contact, and a "fogginess." Recently she began some self-abusive behavior, including hitting her face with her hands.

   You learn that this is the third daughter of a 33-year-old woman. The pregnancy, labor, and delivery were without incident. Her birth weight was 3,200 grams and the Apgar scores were normal. A normal head circumference of 35 cm was obtained. Early developmental milestones were met on time, including smiling, rolling over, sitting up, and walking.

   As the parents recall, things started to change after her first birthday, in the weeks after her third immunization series. She made less and less eye contact, and often seemed to ignore both her parents and sisters. Intake notes indicate that conversations with their family physician led to the impression that their daughter has early signs of probable autism. Noting that they have no related family history, the parents have become increasingly concerned that the immunizations caused some form of brain injury to their child.

At the appointment to see you, your nurse notes that obtaining a respiratory rate was difficult since the child had frequent respiratory pauses. He found a weight and height around the 20th percentile, but a head circumference at the 5th percentile (43 cm).

When you see the child you note she has no dysmorphic features, but her visual attention suggests a lack of interest in her surroundings. The child looks blankly ahead and shows little interest in what you are doing. Her cranial nerves are normal. You note diffuse hypotonia with depressed but present tendon reflexes. Although her age and attentiveness preclude formal muscle testing, the accelerations and velocities of her frequent, restless, antigravity movements suggest normal power. She would not reach for objects or grasp objects placed in her hands. Her gait was wide-based and unsteady.

**What do you do now?**

## RETT SYNDROME

There are multiple clues to the diagnosis here. The rapid developmental decline after 1 year of age, deceleration in head circumference, abnormal breathing pattern, and loss of purposeful movements of the hands in a girl makes Rett syndrome highly probable.

As a first step, therefore, you recommend genetic testing for deletions in the *MECP2* gene (methyl cytosine binding protein 2), which is found on the X chromosome. The *MECP2* gene protein acts as an upstream genetic switch that causes other genes to stop producing their own unique proteins. The genetic defect appears to result in a loss of function of the *MECP2* protein, although the exact mechanism by which the abnormal protein leads to the constellation of findings in Rett syndrome is unknown. MECP2 mutation is a leading cause of severe intellectual impairment in females, and over 90% of girls meeting clinical criteria for Rett syndrome have the MECP2 genetic mutation detected. Other cases may be caused by mutations in nonexpressed, regulatory components of the gene, or by genes that have not yet been identified.

Rett syndrome is a childhood neurodevelopmental disorder characterized by normal early development followed by loss of purposeful use of the hands, slowed brain and head growth, gait abnormalities, seizures, and intellectual impairment. Historically, it was first recognized in females, although a male form of Rett syndrome, typically with profound impairment, also occurs.

The course of Rett syndrome, including the age of onset and the severity of symptoms, varies from child to child, in part as a function of differing patterns of X chromosome inactivation in different patients. Before the symptoms begin, typically in the second year of life, the child appears to grow and develop normally. Then, gradually, mental and physical symptoms appear. Hypotonia (loss of muscle tone) is usually the first symptom. As the syndrome progresses, the child loses purposeful use of her hands and the ability to speak. Early symptoms may include problems crawling or walking. The loss of social skills (diminished eye contact) and repetitive hand movements often lead to a diagnosis of autism before the fact of Rett syndrome is recognized. Loss of functional use of the hands is followed by compulsive hand movements such as wringing and washing, sometimes progressing over weeks or months. Apraxia (the inability to perform motor functions), is perhaps the most severely disabling feature of Rett syndrome, interfering with every body movement, including eye gaze and speech.

Individuals with Rett syndrome often exhibit autistic-like behaviors in the early stages. Many girls with Rett syndrome show intense visual fixation, which is puzzling in terms of their low communication levels. Other symptoms may include toe walking, sleep problems, wide-based gait, teeth grinding, difficulty chewing, slowed growth, and seizures. Breathing signs and symptoms include hyperventilation, apnea (breath-holding), and air swallowing. Table 18.1 lists essential, supportive but not required, and exclusionary features of Rett syndrome.

TABLE 18.1 **Criteria Used in the Diagnosis and Exclusion of Rett Syndrome**

| Essential | Supportive but Not Required | Exclusion |
|---|---|---|
| Normal development until age 6–18 months | Breathing difficulties | Enlargement of body organs or other signs of storage disease |
| Normal head circumference at birth followed by a slowing of the rate of head growth with age (between 3 months and 4 years) | EEG abnormalities Seizures Muscle rigidity, spasticity, and/or joint contracture that worsen with age Decreased mobility with age Scoliosis Teeth grinding Small feet in relation to height | Vision loss due to retinal disorder or optic atrophy Microcephaly at birth An identifiable metabolic disorder or other inherited degenerative disorder |
| Severely impaired expressive language | Growth retardation Decreased body fat and muscle mass | An acquired neurological disorder resulting from severe infection or head trauma |
| Repetitive hand movements | Abnormal sleep patterns Irritability or agitation | |
| Toe walking or an unsteady, wide-based, stiff-legged gait | Chewing and/or swallowing difficulties Poor circulation of the lower extremities, with cold and bluish-red feet and legs Constipation | Evidence of growth retardation in utero or evidence of brain damage acquired after birth |

Some of these clinical features may be age-related.

Four stages of Rett syndrome have been described. Stage I typically begins between 6 and 18 months of age (Since this is a period when infants undergo frequent vaccination, there is often an attribution of the developmental problem to vaccination, as there may be in a variety of neurodevelopmental difficulties). Epidemiological studies however do not support the contention that immunization causes any form of autism. In stage I, reduced eye contact and interest in toys and the surroundings become apparent. Decreased engagement with previously attained milestones such as crawling, sitting, standing, or walking is observed. This stage usually lasts for a few months but can persist for more than a year. Stage II, between ages 1 and 4, may have either a rapid or a gradual onset; purposeful hand skills and spoken language are lost. The characteristic hand movements begin to emerge: wringing, rubbing, clapping, or tapping. Breathing irregularities such as episodes of apnea and hyperventilation may occur. Loss of social interaction and communication may occur. The gait is unsteady, with poor initiation of movement. Slowing of head growth is usually noticed during this stage. Stage III (*plateau*) typically begins between ages 2 and 10 and can last for years. Apraxia, motor problems, and seizures are prominent during this stage, often with reductions in irritability, crying, and autistic-like features. Many girls remain in this stage for most of their lives. Stage IV (*late motor deterioration*) can last for years or decades and is characterized by reduced mobility, weakness, rigidity (stiffness), spasticity, and dystonia. Girls ambulating before this stage may become wheelchair-bound. Usually there is no decline in cognition or communication skills during this phase. Repetitive hand movements may decrease, and eye gaze usually improves.

There is no cure for Rett syndrome, although reversal of pathologic phenotypes has been achieved in some mouse models. Seizures are common in Rett syndrome, and antiepileptic drug therapy may be indicated. Interictal EEG often shows rhythmic slowing, with focal and generalized spike and spike-wave discharges. Since patients with Rett syndrome generally have abnormal EEGs, EEG monitoring is often required in order to differentiate stereotypic, self-injurious, or other repetitive behaviors from definitive epileptic seizures.

> **KEY POINTS TO REMEMBER**
> - The patient develops normally during the first 6 to 18 months of age.
> - Head circumference is normal at birth, with a postnatal deceleration in head growth.
> - Severerly impaired expressive language occurs in all patients.
> - Repetitive, nonpurposeful hand movements are common.
> - Toe walking or an unsteady, wide-based, stiff-legged gait

Further Reading

Axelrod FB, Chelimsky GG, Weese-Mayer DE. Pediatric autonomic disorders. *Pediatrics* 2006;118:309–21.

Chahrour M, Zoghbi HY. The story of Rett syndrome: from clinic to neurobiology. *Neuron* 2007;56:422–37.

Chapleau CA, Lane J, Pozzo-Miller L, Percy AK. Evaluation of current pharmacological treatment options in the management of Rett syndrome: from the present to future therapeutic alternatives. *Curr Clin Pharmacol* 2013;8(4):358–69.

Glaze DG, Frost JD, Jr., Zoghbi HY, Percy AK. Rett's syndrome. Characterization of respiratory patterns and sleep. *Ann Neurol* 1987;21:377–82.

Jedele KB. The overlapping spectrum of Rett and Angelman syndromes: a clinical review. *Semin Pediatr Neurol* 2007;14:108–17.

Liyanage VR, Rastegar M. Rett syndrome and MeCP2. *Neuromol Med* 2014;16(2):231–64. doi:10.1007/s12017-014-8295-9.

Lyst MJ, Bird A. Rett syndrome: a complex disorder with simple roots. *Nature Rev Genetics* 2015;16:261–75.

Matijevic T, Knezevic J, Slavica M, Pavelic J. Rett syndrome: from the gene to the disease. *Eur Neurol* 2009;61:3–10.

Percy AK. Genetics of Rett syndrome: properties of the newly discovered gene and pathobiology of the disorder. *Curr Opin Pediatr* 2000;12:589–95.

Percy AK. Neurobiology and neurochemistry of Rett syndrome. *Eur Child Adolesc Psychiatry* 1997;6(Suppl 1):80–2.

Percy AK. Rett syndrome. *Curr Opin Neurol* 1995;8:156–60.

Williamson SL, Christodoulou J. Rett syndrome: new clinical and molecular insights. *Eur J Hum Genet* 2006;14:896–903.

# 19 The Weak Baby

You are asked by a pediatrician to see a 3-month-old boy with "floppiness." The child was the product of a difficult delivery that ended in a cesarean section because of failure to progress. The mother has two other children in good health, and notes that there were decreased fetal movements compared to her other pregnancies. The full-term infant had moderate respiratory distress at birth but responded well to bag-mask ventilation, and was sent to the well-baby nursery. The mother states that the child has been floppy since birth and she has given up trying to breastfeed him because of a poor latch and suck. Over the past month the parents have become increasingly concerned about his poor head control and muscle tone.

When you see the child you find he has a head circumference (41 cm) and length (62 cm) at the 50th percentile, but a weight (4.8 kg) that is below the 3rd percentile. You find the child to be alert, and no dysmorphic features are present. The child follows a toy with his eyes in all directions. No nystagmus is noted. There appears to be mild bilateral facial weakness. Fasciculations of the tongue (worm-like movements) are noted and the gag is weak. The child has some low-amplitude (short excursion) movements of the hands and feet but has little movement of the arms and legs. Reflexes cannot be elicited. The tone is remarkably decreased, and the head falls back into a full, passive hyperextension when the child is pulled from the supine to the sitting position. Moro reflex is absent.

**What do you do now?**

## SPINAL MUSCULAR ATROPHY

This is obviously a very severe condition. The child's visual alertness and tracking make cerebral pathology an unlikely cause for the hypotonia. The decreased tone and areflexia indicate pathological localization at the anterior horn, peripheral nerve, or muscle. The tongue fasciculations in a young infant are strongly indicative of anterior horn cell disease. The age of presentation and the findings on the neurological examination, taken together, would best fit the diagnosis of spinal muscular atrophy (SMA).

The differential diagnosis would include a number of other disorders of the motor unit. Polyneuropathies are an unusual cause of hypotonia in infants. Among these, congenital hypomyelinating neuropathy can be indistinguishable from infantile SMA. These children typically have EMG findings consistent with denervation and motor nerve conduction velocities that are less than 10 m/sec.

Infantile botulism results from eating food contaminated by an exotoxin of *Clostridium botulinum*. The infants can present with profound hypotonia, ptosis, facial and pharyngeal weakness, dilated pupils, and respiratory failure. Typically there is a prodromal syndrome of constipation and poor feeding. In this case the decreased fetal movements and poor tone present from birth would indicate a congenital rather than an acquired disorder.

Congenital (genetically based) or autoimmune (transplacentally transmitted antibody) myasthenia gravis may present with hypotonia. Mothers with myasthenia gravis may deliver a baby with transient weakness due to passive transfer of acetylcholine receptor antibodies to the fetus. Less often, infants from a healthy mother harboring an antibody to the acetylcholine receptor may present with hypotonia or joint contractures at birth. Familial infantile myasthenia presents with prominent respiratory and feeding difficulties at birth, whereas congenital myasthenia gravis has ophthalmoplegia as the primary clinical picture. Unlike myasthenia gravis seen in older children and adults, congenital myasthenia, most often recessively inherited, is not caused by an autoimmune process but results from genetic mutations affecting transmission at the neuromuscular junction. Mutations in a variety of genes have been identified. A decremental EMG response on low-frequency stimulation of the compound muscle action potential can be seen.

A number of congenital myopathies can present with neonatal hypotonia and weakness. Congenital myotonic dystrophy presents with pronounced facial diplegia with a tent-shaped mouth, arthrogryposis, hypotonia, and weakness. The clinical features of congenital myotonic dystrophy are typically more severe than SMA in the neonatal period. Other congenital myopathies such as central core disease, multiminicore disease, myotubular myopathy, and nemaline myopathy typically have only mild hypotonia at birth and are usually diagnosed at a later age.

SMA is the most common lethal genetic disorder of infancy, affecting approximately one in 10,000 live births. The disorder is characterized by symmetrical proximal muscle weakness and is caused by a degeneration of the anterior horn cells of the spinal cord, although other neuronal subpopulations in the motor system are also affected. SMA is classically divided into three types based on age of onset and clinical manifestations, although the subtypes actually fall on a continuum. The most severe type (SMA I, also called Werdnig-Hoffman disease) always begins before 6 months of age, and these infants typically never sit independently; the intermediate type (SMA II) begins between 6 and 18 months, and patients may, at least temporarily, attain independent sitting; the juvenile type (SMA III) begins after 18 months, and some patients attain independent walking.

SMA is associated with homozygous mutations in the survival motor neuron 1 gene (SMN1) and its centromeric homolog, SMN2. The genes lie within the telomeric and centromeric halves of a large inverted repeat in chromosome 5q13. In this autosomal recessive condition, there is usually no prior family history of SMA. The parents may each be found to have one normal copy of the gene and one mutant copy. The tissue selectivity of this ubiquitously expressed protein in the setting of SMA remains puzzling, especially since it is involved in fundamental aspects of RNA metabolism. Approximately one in 50 to one in 200 people worldwide carry a mutation of the SMN1 gene. Therefore, considering the severity of this disease, identification of the SMN1 deletion in a proband can have important genetic counseling implications for ostensible carriers of this mutation.

In this case, since the child is not critically ill, the first step is to obtain genetic testing for mutations of the *SMN1* gene. While EMG and nerve conduction studies would be useful in differentiating SMA from botulism, myotonic dystrophy, and a polyneuropathy, there is little reason to do these studies unless the genetic test, which is more than 95% sensitive in the setting of type I SMA, returns normal. Unfortunately, in this child, there were zero copies of the *SMN1* gene and only two copies of the *SMN2* gene; an increased number (at least three copies) of *SMN2* has been associated with a less severe phenotype of SMA.

Because there is no effective therapy for SMA, management consists of preventing or treating the complications of severe weakness, such as restrictive lung disease, poor nutrition, orthopedic deformities, immobility, and psychosocial problems.

> **KEY POINTS TO REMEMBER**
> - SMA is a disorder of the anterior horn cell characterized by hypotonia, weakness, and areflexia
> - SMA is not associated with dysmorphism or abnormalities of other organs
> - Subtype delineation of SMA depends primarily on age of onset.
> - All patients with SMA have progressive disease, although survival into the second decade can occur in type 1 SMA.

Further Reading

Arnold WD, Kassar D, Kissel JT. Spinal muscular atrophy: diagnosis and management in a new therapeutic era. *Muscle Nerve* 2015;51:157–67.

Darras BT. Spinal muscular atrophies. *Pediatr Clin North Am* 2015;62:743–66.

Johnston HM. The floppy weak infant revisited. *Brain Dev* 2003;25:155–8.

Lorson CL, Rindt H, Shababi M. Spinal muscular atrophy: Mechanisms and therapeutic strategies. *Human Mol Genet* 2010;19:R111–8.

Markowitz JA, Tinkle MB, Fischbeck KH. Spinal muscular atrophy in the neonate. *J Obstet Gynecol Neonatal Nurs* 2004;33:12–20.

Ogino S, Wilson RB. Genetic testing and risk assessment for spinal muscular atrophy (SMA). *Hum Genet* 2002;111:477–500.

Prior TW. Perspectives and diagnostic considerations in spinal muscular atrophy. *Genet Med* 2010;12:145–52.

Russman BS. Spinal muscular atrophy: clinical classification and disease heterogeneity. *J Child Neurol* 2007;22:946–51.

Tisdale S, Pellizzoni L. Disease mechanisms and therapeutic approaches in spinal muscular atrophy. *J Neurosci* 2015;35:8691–700.

# 20 Contents Under Pressure

The pediatrician calling you is seeing a 2-year-old girl in his office who has been having episodes of early morning vomiting for most of the past month. The child is well known to the pediatrician, who has been following her since birth. She tells you that the girl was born after an uneventful pregnancy, labor, and spontaneous vaginal delivery, with normal Apgar scores, birthweight, length, and head circumference. The girl's routine office visits were uneventful.

Three weeks ago the parents noted the girl began having episodes of early morning emesis. They would hear her gagging and frequently find her in a pool of vomitus. The child would tell the parents that both her stomach and head hurt during the event.

The pediatrician describes the child as being alert and active. Her general and neurological examinations were considered normal. However, of concern to the pediatrician is that the girl's head circumference is above the 95th percentile. She wonders whether the child may have an intracranial tumor.

**What do you do now?**

## HYDROCEPHALUS

Macrocephaly, "large head," is commonly defined as two standard deviations above the normal population. This definition indicates that 2% of the normal population has macrocephaly, and many of these are benign, or constitutional. The history of morning emesis warrants prompt evaluation. Increased intracranial pressure can result in emesis, particularly in the morning, which may be due to lying flat during the night, circadian hormonal changes, or some combination of these (lying flat increases intracranial pressure, whereas standing or sitting reduces intracranial pressure).

To assess the probability of a connection between the apparent macrocrania and the morning vomiting, you ask the pediatrician what her head circumference percentiles have been historically. A simple graph, the head circumference growth curve, depicting growth velocity of the occipitofrontal circumference since birth, will help to distinguish between a scenario of chronic/congenital versus acquired macrocrania. In this case the child's head circumference growth velocity has in fact accelerated such that when measured at age 2, she was near the 60th percentile, whereas now she is above the 98th percentile. This makes it very likely that some acquired, space-occupying lesion, either a tumor or hydrocephalus, has progressed to the point of causing the morning symptoms in this child. Therefore, the next step would be to obtain an MRI to rule out hydrocephalus or a structural lesion or other cause of acquired macrocrania.

Meanwhile, since even some toddlers with (temporarily) high head growth velocity may have familial macrocrania (and, incidentally, a period of high head growth velocity occurs in many cases of autism), it will also be appropriate to measure the head circumferences of the parents. One might be at least partially reassured about the intracranial hypertension question if both of the parents had head circumferences above the 95th percentile. When you measure the head circumferences of the parents, you note that these measurements are both normal, making a benign constitutional/familial cause of the elevated head circumference in this child less likely.

Besides tumor, the pathological causes of macrocephaly are many and include both chronic/congenital (autism, neurofibromatosis type 1, hydrocephalus, thickening of the skull) and other acquired (secondary hydrocephalus, intracranial hemorrhage) conditions. Neuroimaging, preferably

MRI, is generally required to sort out whether a child has macrocrania on the basis of excess *extra-axial* intracranial tissue (Table 20.1) versus megalencephaly (large brain). Megalencephaly represents a subset of children with macrocephaly in whom the brain is enlarged, and this also may be either a familial/benign or constitutional, or a pathological, condition (e.g., storage disorders; Table 20.2).

The MRI shows hydrocephalus: there is enlargement of the lateral and third ventricle, with a normal fourth ventricle (Fig. 20–1). Hydrocephalus is divided into two types, communicating (nonobstructive) or noncommunicating (obstructive), depending on whether cerebrospinal fluid communicates between the ventricles and subarachnoid space. In addition to morning vomiting and increasing head circumference, either type may present with headache, weight loss, sleepiness, high-pitched cry, or failure to thrive. On physical examination of infants with hydrocephalus, one typically sees a bulging fontanel, splayed sutures, enlarged head, and "sunset" sign (deviation of the eyes downward).

In this case, the findings are indicative of communicating hydrocephalus. Aqueductal stenosis is eliminated as a possibility because the fourth ventricle is enlarged. Figure 20–2 is an example of a patient with foramen of Monro obstruction with unilateral ventricular enlargement. At this point the patient should be referred to neurosurgery for possible shunt placement.

TABLE 20.1 **Causes of Macrocrania *Without* Megalencephaly**

| Disorder | Comments |
| --- | --- |
| Hydrocephalus | Wide variety of underlying congenital and acquired disorders, and anatomic subtypes (communicating/noncommunicating). Common complication of intraventricular hemorrhage in the setting of prematurity. |
| Tumor | Location of tumor (on neuroimaging) often a clue to pathology, |
| Blood | Most often associated with trauma or catastrophic bleed, |
| Cranioskeletal disorders | Physical exam often shows dysmorphism. |

TABLE 20.2 **Causes of Megalencephaly**

| Disorder | Comments |
| --- | --- |
| Achondroplasia | Autosomal dominant genetic disorder; dwarfism; large skull and brain. Also may be associated with (obstructive) hydrocephalus. |
| Autism | Many cases with no defined etiology have macrocephaly in common. |
| Alexander disease | An autosomal dominant disease with megalencephaly, seizures, spasticity, dementia, and occasional hydrocephalus. It is caused by mutations in the gene for glial fibrillary acidic protein (GFAP) that maps to chromosome 17q21. |
| Canavan disease | An autosomal recessive leukodystrophy with degeneration of myelin and megalencephaly. |
| Epidermal nevus syndrome | A neurocutaneous syndrome associated with epidermal nevus and seizures, spasticity, mental retardation, and developmental delay. Hydrocephalus may occur. |
| Gangliosidosis | Lipid storage disorder caused by the accumulation of lipids. Associated with megalencephaly. |
| Glutaric aciduria | An inherited disorder in which lysine, hydroxylysine, and tryptophan cannot be metabolized; excessive levels of their intermediate breakdown products (glutaric acid) result in neurological dysfunction. Megalencephaly is common. |
| Hypomelanosis of Ito | Condition with large, hypopigmented area that is whorled or streaked, seizures, mental retardation, and megalencephaly. |
| Incontinentia pigmenti | Condition associated with swirling macular hyperpigmentation or linear hypopigmentation, mental retardation, seizures, megalencephaly |
| Krabbe disease | Autosomal recessive metabolic disorder due to the absence or marked reduction of galactocerebrosidase, which can lead to megalencephaly, seizures, developmental delay. |
| Maple syrup urine disease | Autosomal recessive metabolic disorder of branched-chain amino acids; poor feeding, vomiting, dehydration, lethargy, hypotonia, seizures, ketoacidosis, pancreatitis, coma. |

(*continued*)

TABLE 20.2 **Continued**

| Disorder | Comments |
| --- | --- |
| Metachromatic leukodystrophy | Leukodystrophy with abnormal myelin due to sulfatide accumulation. |
| Neurofibromatosis (type 1) | Autosomal dominant—megalencephaly, intellectual impairment, café-au-lait spots. Autosomal dominant. |
| Mucopolysaccharidoses | Lysosomal disorder; impaired degradation of glycosaminoglycans. Cognitive impairment. |
| Sotos syndrome | Excessive physical growth during the first 2–3 years of life. Associated with mental retardation, delayed motor, cognitive, and social development, hypotonia (low muscle tone), speech impairments. |
| Tuberous sclerosis | Neurocutaneous disorder with cerebral tubers, seizures, mental retardation |

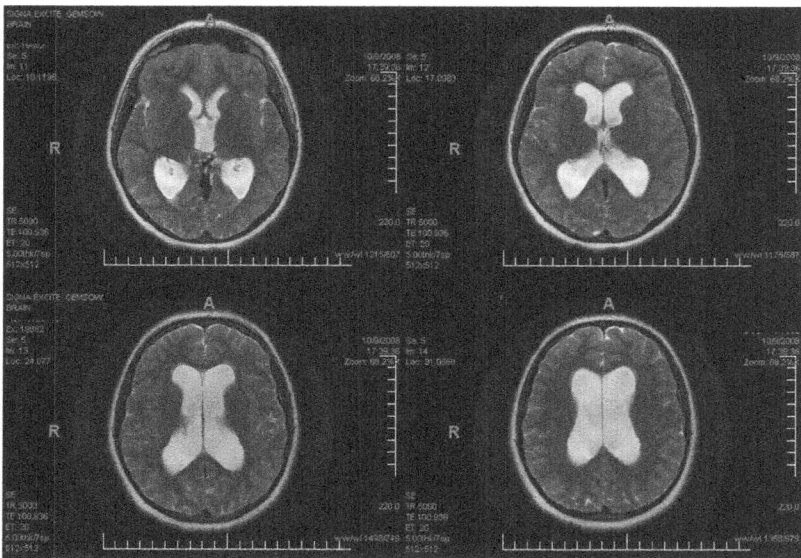

**FIGURE 20-1** MRI from a 2-year-old with communicating hydrocephalus. The fourth ventricle, which is not shown here, is also enlarged, indicating that the four ventricles communicate with each other.

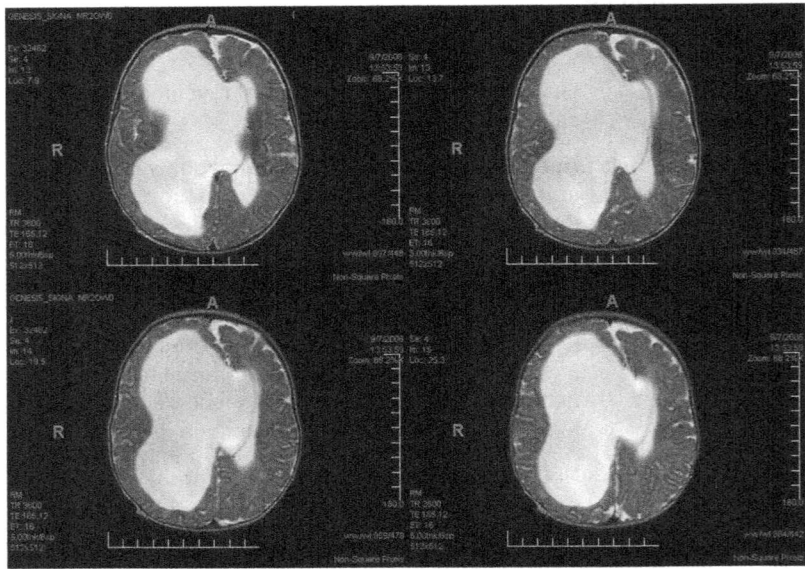

**FIGURE 20-2** Unilateral left hemisphere hydrocephalus due to obstruction of the foramen of Monro.

The history and physical examination in the setting of hydrocephalus may also disclose clues to differentiate *extrinsic* (e.g., postmeningitis, posthemorrhagic, among other causes) from *intrinsic* (e.g., L1CAM mutation, a cause of congenital, X-linked hydrocephalus, with adducted thumbs) causes of hydrocephalus. Hydrocephalus, accompanying Chiari malformation, is common in the setting of neural tube defects. Other syndromes featuring hydrocephalus include craniosynostoses and dysmorphologic syndromes (Noonan syndrome, VACTERL, others).

> **KEY POINTS TO REMEMBER**
> - Hydrocephalus may present with vomiting, headache, weight loss
> - Sunsetting, with downward deviation of the eyes, can be a sign of hydrocephalus.
> - MRI will differentiate hydrocephaly from megalencephaly of other etiologies.

Further Reading

Bhattacharyya KB, Senapati A, Basu S, et al. Bobble-head doll syndrome: some atypical features with a new lesion and review of the literature. *Acta Neurol Scand* 2003;108:216–320.

Hommet C, Billard C, Gillet P, et al. Neuropsychologic and adaptive functioning in adolescents and young adults shunted for congenital hydrocephalus. *J Child Neurol* 1999;14:144–150.

McAllister JP. Pathophysiology of congenital and neonatal hydrocephalus. *Semin Fetal Neonatal Med* 2012;17:285–294.

Tully HM, Dobyns WB. Infantile hydrocephalus: A review of epidemiology, classification and causes. *Eur J Med Genet* 2014;57:359–368.

Shemie S, Jay V, Rutka J, Armstrong D. Acute obstructive hydrocephalus and sudden death in children. *Ann Emerg Med* 1997;29(4):524–528.

# 21 Episodic Weakness: Seeing Through the Smoke

You are called about a 5-year-old girl who is being transferred to the pediatric intensive care unit (PICU) from another hospital with episodes of transient left-sided weakness involving the face and arm. The episodes would occur multiple times daily, last 4 to 5 minutes, and then clear totally. The PICU attendings tell you the neurological examination appears normal. A CT scan of the head from the outside hospital was also normal.

Considering the possibility that these episodes were seizures, the PICU staff ordered an EEG. The EEG showed some right-sided slowing but no epileptiform activity. During hyperventilation the patient developed an episode of left-sided weakness that lasted approximately 5 minutes and then cleared. The child was able to talk throughout the episode. During the left-sided hemiparesis the EEG showed high-amplitude slowing that persisted for 5 minutes beyond the end of hyperventilation. The PICU staff asks for advice.

When you see the child, you learn from the parents that she has been having episodes for about 4 months. Since the girl seemed to improve relatively quickly after the attacks, the parents decided these changes could have been part of normal play. Their concern increased when the attacks increased in frequency, and even more since that the child now seems to have persistent left-sided weakness. On examination, the child is inattentive, limiting the formal motor power testing. Cranial nerve examination shows subtle flattening of the left nasalobial fold, and on observational motor examination flexor posturing of the left arm, a left-sided pyramidal sign, appears in stressed gait sequences (toe walking, walking on the lateral edge of the foot). The examination is otherwise unremarkable, with normal visual fields, extraocular muscle movements, and cerebellar function.

### What do you do now?

## MOYAMOYA DISEASE

Although "inhibitory" partial seizures remain a possibility, it is unusual for children to develop weakness as the sole manifestation of the seizures. Most seizures result in "positive" symptomatology with tonic, clonic, or myoclonic activity during the event rather than weakness. Conceivably the child is having partial motor seizures that were overlooked, with postictal weakness (Todd's paralysis).

Another consideration would be alternating hemiplegia of childhood. Children with alternating hemiplegia typically are developmentally delayed and have abnormal neurological examinations. As indicated by the name, the motor impairment alternates between sides. This is an unlikely diagnosis in this case, however, because alternating hemiplegia has its onset before 18 months of age and this patient's weakness has been consistently on the left side of the body. Periodic paralysis (hyperkalemic, hypokalemic, or normokalemic) may result in episodic weakness, although it is unusual for it to involve only one side of the body.

The persistent high-voltage slowing during the EEG and onset of symptoms during hyperventilation raise the possibility of a neurovascular, ischemic cause. Hyperventilation during EEG is contraindicated in children with sickle cell disease, for example, because the hypocarbia may exacerbate a baseline cerebrovascular stenosis and precipitate brain ischemia, which registers as high-voltage slowing on the EEG. Hyperventilation effectively reduces $PCO_2$ and cerebral blood flow, resulting in signs and symptoms due to ischemia. Another potential underlying neurovascular lesion that may make the child's brain vulnerable to hyperventilation is Moyamoya disease. Onset of symptoms in this patient during hyperventilation prompts you to suggest MRI with MRI angiography. This shows the vascular pathology, and related parenchymal signal change, characteristic of this cerebrovascular syndrome.

Moyamoya represents a cerebrovascular condition that may occur in a variety of settings. The clinical features include cerebral ischemia (strokes), recurrent transient ischemic attacks, sensorimotor paralysis (numbness in the extremities), convulsions, and/or migraine-like headaches. Cerebrovascular occlusion of the internal carotid artery, once it begins, tends to continue despite any known medical management. In some people this leads to repeated strokes and severe functional impairment or even death. In others, the blockage may not cause any symptoms.

This is a chronic, progressive, noninflammatory vasculopathy that results in a slow occlusion of the intracranial arteries, causing a successive ischemic event. Hemorrhagic events can also occur, especially later in the course of the disorder. The occlusion typically begins at the carotid siphon. The condition leads to irreversible blockage of the carotid arteries to the brain as they enter the skull. It affects either children (although more often adolescents) or adults, where strokes are often both cortical and subcortical in distribution. In children it tends to cause strokes or seizures; presentations in adults more often feature hemorrhagic strokes.

Because the occlusion is slowly progressive, multiple anastomoses form between the internal and external carotid arteries. The diagnosis is initially suggested by CT, MRI, or angiogram. The definitive diagnosis is based on conventional angiography, where these anastomoses result in an appearance of a "puff of smoke." This angiographic appearance of multiple compensatory dilated striate vessels (Fig. 21–1) is how Moyamoya loosely translates from Japanese. Contrast-enhanced MRI T1-weighted images are

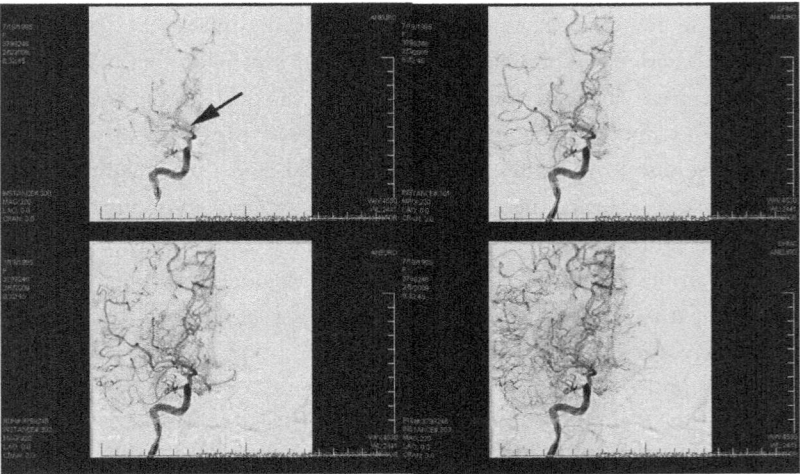

**FIGURE 21–1** Cerebral arteriogram from a 10-year-old girl showing severe stenosis of the supraclinoid internal carotid artery (*arrow*). Collateral flow to the peripheral anterior and middle cerebral arteries is supplied by lenticulostriate collaterals, leptomeningeal branches from the posterior cerebral artery, and transdural anastomoses from the ophthalmic artery.

better than FLAIR images for depicting the leptomeningeal "ivy sign" in Moyamoya disease. MRI and MRI angiography should be performed at the time of diagnosis and for follow-up of Moyamoya disease. In some centers, nuclear medicine studies such as SPECT (single-photon emission computed tomography) are used to demonstrate the decreased blood and oxygen supply to areas of the brain involved with Moyamoya disease. Diffusion-weighted MRI can also be used to follow the clinical course of Moyamoya disease in children who develop new deficits.

Moyamoya can be either familial or acquired. Patients with Down syndrome, neurofibromatosis, or sickle cell disease, among other conditions, seem to be at increased risk for developing Moyamoya malformations. Brain radiation therapy in children is a risk factor for the condition. The gene responsible for familial Moyamoya disease is on chromosome 17q25. Patients should be evaluated for an underlying vasculopathy or coagulopathy. Neurovascular surgical treatment options include surgical bypass procedures.

> **KEY POINTS TO REMEMBER**
> - Often presents with quick onset and offset of hemiparesis
> - Unlike alternating hemiplegia, typically involves one side of the body, and presents at an older age
> - Persistent unilateral slowing on the EEG following hyperventilation suggests the disorder.
> - Consultation with a pediatric neurosurgeon specializing in neurovascular disease is in order.

Further Reading

Ausman JI, Diaz FG, Ma SH, et al. Cerebrovascular occlusive disease in children: a survey. *Acta Neurochir (Wien)* 1988;94:117–28.

Currie S. Childhood Moyamoya disease and Moyamoya syndrome: a pictorial review. *Pediatr Neurol* 2011;44:401–13.

Giroud M, Lemesle M, Madinier G, et al. Stroke in children under 16 years of age. Clinical and etiological difference with adults. *Acta Neurol Scand* 1997;96:401–6.

Kitahara T, Ariga N, Yamaura A, et al. Familial occurrence of moyamoya disease: report of three Japanese families. *J Neurol Neurosurg Psychiatry* 1979;42:208–14.

Rafay MF, Armstrong D, Dirks P, et al. Patterns of cerebral ischemia in children with Moyamoya. *Pediatr Neurol* 2015;52:65–72.

Ullrich NJ, Robertson R, Kinnamon DD, et al. Moyamoya following cranial irradiation for primary brain tumors in children. *Neurology* 2007;68:932–8.

Yamashiro Y, Takahashi H, Takahashi K. Cerebrovascular Moyamoya disease. *Eur J Pediatr* 1984;142:44–50.

# SECTION III

# Potpourri: Inflammatory, Pain, Neuropsychiatric, and Movement Disorders

# 22  A Panoply of Symptoms

A 10-year-old girl comes in because of personality change. The course started 6 weeks ago when, one morning, and for the following day and 2 weeks, her parents noted that she seemed to have a limp and to be dragging her right foot. At first her parents thought she was imitating a character she had seen on television. During this time she also had some trouble with her handwriting and reaching and grasping things with her right arm and hand. As these motor problems seemed to persist, the parents were about to contact the child's physician— but then they seemed to abate and almost disappeared at the end of 2 weeks. Although her speech never fully improved, her parents decided to put off calling the doctor.

Then, just as the motor symptoms were waning, the child started to become increasingly angry and irritable. She pushed her younger brother, with whom she was normally friendly and protective, while they were brushing their teeth one morning in the bathroom. Then she was so regretful that she cried through the morning and stayed home from school. She was sullen and refused to spend time with her friends, whom she now mistrusted.

On further history she has had no other systemic symptoms, but her parents do note that intermittently, her left, or possibly her right, eye seems to turn in. Her appetite may have increased somewhat, although her weight has been stable. On examination you confirm a sullen, passive, or withdrawn affect. Her cranial nerves appear normal, although ocular her smooth pursuit movements appear fragmented. Motor exam is the most telling: she has slowing of rapid alternating movements on the right, mild (4+) grip weakness on the right, and some flexor posturing of the right arm when asked to perform a stressed gait maneuver ("Walk on the outside edges of your feet, please"). Her general physical examination is otherwise unremarkable.

Considering these objective signs, and the possibility of a brain tumor, you decide to carry out a head MRI the same day, with and without gadolinium contrast. The result is that she has four different nonenhancing T2 bright areas, centered in the gray matter, and crossing over known vascular territories of the brain: three in the left hemisphere, partially extending into subjacent white matter, and one on the right. There are no lesions below the tentorium.

**What do you do now?**

## NMDA RECEPTOR AB ENCEPHALOPATHY

The child has a global encephalopathy with fluctuating motor signs. The head MRI does not suggest a neoplasm or a cerebrovascular disorder, and neither the time course nor the imaging suggests a metabolic or a degenerative brain condition. Inflammatory or dysimmune brain pathologies appear most likely in this case, and the one that has received the most attention over the past few decades would be acute disseminated encephalomyelitis (ADEM). However, two considerations weigh *against* this (relatively heterogeneous) condition: first, she never really showed encephalopathy in the sense of a depressed mental status (confusion, lethargy) and altered mental status is considered one of the central diagnostic criteria for ADEM; second, the MRI lesions conspicuously involve the gray matter of the cerebrum. Although some degree of "spilling over" of white matter lesions on MRI in ADEM can be seen, it would be rare to see this much gray matter involvement in that condition.

The conditions and associated key laboratory findings that may feature MRI findings such as the present case are outlined in Table 22.1.

You perform a lumbar puncture, which proves normal. Blood and CSF are sent for NMDA receptor antibody testing. Ten days later, these tests return positive in CSF but negative in blood. The child is put on a moderate dose (2 mg/kg/day) of prednisone. Over the following weeks, her mood improves, and her persisting dysarthria and intermittent strabismus also remit. Abdominal ultrasound and CT scan, to assess for the possibility of an occult ovarian neoplasm, are normal. Three months later a follow-up MRI scan shows just a trace of two of the former T2 bright abnormalities, and the child has a normal neurological examination. She continues to do well over the course of an ensuing 2-month gradual taper of the prednisone and during continuing yearly follow-up clinic visits.

NMDA receptor encephalitis is likely a widely underrecognized cause of subacute or acute neurological symptoms, including seizures or an encephalitis-like picture, and it appears to have a seasonal pattern of onset in the pediatric age group. This case demonstrates the impact of the serologic test for this disorder on therapeutic decision making and on the clinical course, supporting in turn a high level of suspicion in a fairly diverse array of potential clinical contexts. It is noteworthy that CSF is

TABLE 22.1 **Conditions Featuring Acquired Multifocal, T2 Bright Lesions of the Brain**

| Diagnostic Entity | Laboratory Markers | Therapeutic Considerations |
|---|---|---|
| NMDA receptor antibody encephalitis* | Anti-NMDA-R antibody serology (blood, CSF) | Corticosteroids, other immunomodulatory therapies |
| Lyme disease | Lyme serology (blood, CSF) | Ceftriaxone, doxycycline |
| Microangiopathic vasculitis | ANCA, brain biopsy, DADA mutation | Corticosteroids, other immunomodulatory therapies |
| Multiple sclerosis/ADEM | Oligoclonal bands | Corticosteroids |
| Viral encephalitides | Viral serology (blood, CSF) | Supportive care, antiviral agents (HSV) |
| Lupus CNS involvement | ANA | Corticosteroids, other immunomodulatory therapies |

*See discussion regarding other possible immune-mediated encephalitides.

often positive even when serum is negative, emphasizing that a blood test is not adequate to assess for NMDA receptor encephalitis. NMDA receptor encephalitis has also been reported as a sequel to HSV encephalitis. While NMDA receptor antibody encephalitis appears to be the most common type, other immune-mediated encephalitides feature antibodies against a potassium voltage-gated channel and other epitopes of NMDA receptors (AMPA receptor antibodies).

Other manifestations associated with NMDA receptor antibody-mediated encephalitis include focal seizures, and the clinical scope of these presentations is still being defined. It appears that the EEG background may initially be abnormal, with subsequent progressive deterioration of the background EEG as a clue to the underlying dysimmune etiology. Dyskinesias and psychiatric or cognitive symptoms may be presenting or later-emerging symptoms in this heterogeneous disorder. In addition to corticosteroid therapy, rituximab represents an alternate pharmacotherapeutic consideration.

With regard to the possibility of an underlying neoplasm, adults seems to have a higher rate of occult cancers in NMDA receptor antibody neurological syndromes compared to children. Since occult neoplasms in this context have been reported in older adolescents, it is probably wise to perform some screening tests for teratoma, the most commonly identified underlying tumor. Presumably, the tumor stimulates the immune system to generate a pathogenic autoantibody that cross-reacts with brain synapses to a devastating effect.

> **KEY POINTS TO REMEMBER**
>
> - The temporal course may be subacute or fulminant, with conspicuous psychiatric symptoms.
> - MRI findings may be confused with acute disseminated encephalomyelitis or other encephalitides.
> - A high level of suspicion and serologic testing from both CSF and blood are critical to diagnosis.
> - Immunomodulatory therapy, most often with corticosteroids, appears effective
> - Other antibody-mediated syndromes may resemble NMDA Receptor AB encephalopathy: AMPA receptor, ABA-B receptor, LGI1, CASPR2

Further Reading

Adang LA, Lynch DR, Panzer JA. Pediatric anti-NMDA receptor encephalitis is seasonal. *Ann Clin Transl Neurol* 2014;1:921–925.

Dale RC, Brilot F, Duffy LV, et al. Utility and safety of rituximab in pediatric autoimmune and inflammatory CNS disease. *Neurology* 2014;83:142–50.

Dalmau J, Gleichman AJ, Hughes EG, et al. Anti-NMDA-receptor encephalitis: case series and analysis of the effects of antibodies. *Lancet Neurol* 2008;7:1091–8.

Day GS, High SM, Cot B, Tang-Wai DF. Anti-NMDA-receptor encephalitis: case report and literature review of an under-recognized condition. *J Gen Internal Med* 2011;26:811–6.

Krupp LB, Tardieu M, Amato MP, et al. International Pediatric Multiple Sclerosis Study Group criteria for pediatric multiple sclerosis and immune-mediated central nervous system demyelinating disorders: revisions to the 2007 definitions. *Multiple Sclerosis J 2013*;19:1261–7.

Leypoldt F, Armangue T, Dalmau J. Autoimmune encephalopathies. *Ann NY Acad Sci* 2015;1338:94–115.

Lim SY, Panikkath R, Mankongpaisarnrung C, et al. Anti-N-methyl-D-aspartate receptor encephalitis. *Am J Med Sci* 2013;345:491–493.

Sands TT, Nash K, Tong S, Sullivan J. Focal seizures in children with anti-NMDA receptor antibody encephalitis. *Epilepsy Res* 2015;112:31–36.

# 23 The Girl with the Bizarre Gait

When the ER physician calls you about a 14-year-old girl who has presented because of 3 days of progressive gait instability, you can hear the regret in his voice. He is sorry to be calling you, because the girl's blithe affect and bizarre swaying seem to be sure indicators that this child has a functional (psychosomatic) neurological disorder. The referring physician isn't sure what to make of the fact that the patient does have a slightly high resting pulse (110) and blood pressure (136/90).

You arrive to find a pleasant adolescent female resting comfortably. Her father works as a nurse and appears to have an assertive personality, as upon your arrival he demands that his daughter undergo a head MRI—he is concerned that she has a brain tumor. The patient's main complaint is of poor balance—"I feel like the floor is just slipping out from under me." The balance problem has been progressing day by day, and there are no other pointers to neurological problems on historical review of systems. Other than a diarrheal illness that had affected several other family members 2 weeks before, she has been well. Her medical history is benign, and she has no recent travel from her home.

On general examination she does indeed have a high resting pulse and blood pressure. Otherwise her general examination is normal, with a normal range of affect—in fact she is strikingly composed and consistent, and articulate. Her speech is fluent and oriented, and she has normal cranial nerves. Power testing shows some mild proximal weakness in the deltoids (4+), biceps (4+), and intrinsic hand muscles (finger abduction 4+), but when you examine her leg strength her smiling and laughing make you wonder if her effort is full: she seems to have at least grade 4 to 4- strength in all leg muscle groups when tested in supine position. Her reflexes are absent. Sensation to light touch and sharp seem fine, but her position sense is consistently off on both blind finger-touch and sense of passive joint movement ("Am I moving your toe up or down?").

Upon standing, she sways wildly and seems to misreach as she grasps for the bedrail, as both you and her parent move quickly to prevent her falling. A trial of independent walking seems too hazardous.

What do you do now?

## GUILLAIN-BARRÉ SYNDROME

A common issue for pediatric specialists is how to support the referral process of the generalists with whom we work (have we facilitated, or discouraged, referral of patients with suspected psychosomatic disorders?) and concurrently how to avoid the pitfall of becoming cognitively "anchored" in the initial diagnostic impression of that referring clinician. In this case, the referring clinician's error stemmed from overemphasis on (1) the apparent mismatch between the patient's symptoms and her apparent subjective level of concern—was this "la belle indifference" often associated with psychosomatic disorders in adolescents? And (2) the apparent mismatch between her strength and her gait stability, which suggested the possibility of poor effort, also commonly associated with functional neurological disorders. Your findings of hyporeflexia and impaired proprioception represent key objective physical findings in this case, ones that fit with an acute polyneuropathy rather than with a functional neurological disorder.

Possible causes of acute polyneuropathy are outlined in Table 23.1. However, by far the most commonly encountered diagnosis in this context is Guillain-Barré syndrome (GBS), also known as acute polyneuritis. This is the most common cause of acquired paralysis in children. It initially

TABLE 23.1 **Causes of Acute Polyneuropathy**

| | Electrophysiology | Relevant Laboratory Finding |
|---|---|---|
| Tick bite paralysis | Axonal neuropathy | None—careful physical examination for engorged *Dermacentor* tick |
| Heavy metal intoxication | Axonal neuropathy | Blood for heavy metal screen |
| Porphyria | Axonal neuropathy | Urine/blood porphyrins |
| Chemotherapy (vincristine) | Axonal neuropathy | None—exposure history |
| Organophosphate Intoxication | Axonal neuropathy | Red blood cell/plasma cholinesterase activity |

tends to progress over 7 to 14 days, with a more protracted recovery over months.

GBS often presents with pain, which may delay the diagnosis, and it most often presents with symmetrical ascending paralysis with areflexia. Progression over days (less than 1 month) and onset of recovery 2 to 4 weeks after the onset of plateau are supportive of the diagnosis. *Campylobacter jejuni* is the organism most clearly associated with the condition. GBS represents a spectrum of conditions and includes autoimmunity in some cases to the axon as well as the myelin/Schwann cell. Key findings required for diagnosis include progressive motor weakness in at least two limbs and areflexia/hyporeflexia.

Two immediate management questions arise. First, if this is GBS, where should the patient be observed? Considering the possibility of impending neurogenic respiratory failure, a patient with gait problems and known or suspected GBS should in most cases, at least initially, be observed in the hospital or ICU. The second question becomes one of the timing and sequencing of the most useful, initial diagnostic tests: electrophysiological testing and CSF examination. (Although contrast MRI of the lumbar spine for nerve root enhancement or nerve biopsy could also be considered, these are not considered first-line diagnostic tests relative to published diagnostic criteria for GBS.)

Electromyography/nerve conduction velocity will probably show a greater sensitivity when the patient has had symptoms for at least 1 week. Therefore, the most appropriate next step diagnostically for this patient would be a lumbar puncture to assess for "albumino-cytologic dissociation"—the finding, contrasting with the CSF profile seen in poliomyelitis, of elevated protein, with a relatively moderate lymphocytic pleocytosis (typically less than 10 to 20 white blood cells/mm$^3$). This finding (elevated CSF protein) may not occur until after 1 week of symptoms.

You explain to the parent that the findings are compelling for a disorder of the peripheral nervous system, and he acquiesces to your direction that imaging of the central nervous system can be deferred in favor of a lumbar puncture. The patient is found to have a protein level of 66 mg/dL, with 13 lymphocytes/mm$^3$, and a normal opening pressure. She is admitted to the hospital for initiation of intravenous gamma globulin (IVIG) and monitoring of her autonomic and respiratory status with periodic measurements of her pulmonary vital capacity. On day 3 of the hospital stay an EMG shows multifocal slowing of nerve conduction velocities, consistent with the demyelinative process seen in GBS.

Clinical trials in adults show that steroids are not indicated in the treatment of this disorder. Historically, the use of IVIG in pediatrics has been based on extrapolation of studies showing its effectiveness in adults. This treatment probably shortens the course in children with the disease. It is similar in efficacy to plasma exchange, and the combination of the two is probably not more effective than either treatment alone.

The parent asks if any other testing can be done to deduce the ultimate etiology, or trigger, of GBS, now confirmed in his daughter. Medical centers vary in their laboratory testing strategy aimed at identifying a precipitating infectious pathogen in this setting. Although in Lyme-endemic areas, *Borrelia burgdoferi* is reputed to precipitate GBS, the frequency of Lyme seropositivity in these areas is high enough that a chance association may be questioned, and definitive epidemiological evidence supporting a causal association is awaited. Serologic evidence of viral or bacterial enteritides could be considered, but it is not clear, other than perhaps in the case of *C. jejuni* (which sometimes precipitates a severe, axonal variant of GBS), that these tests would alter management.

**KEY POINTS TO REMEMBER**

- Not all ataxia is cerebellar labyrinthine in origin—check position sense.
- Significant signs and symptoms attributable to GBS will be associated with a-reflexia/hypo-reflexia.
- Check spinal fluid for high protein.
- Monitor closely in recent onset GBS.

Further Reading

Asbury AK, Cornblath DR. Assessment of current diagnostic criteria for Guillain-Barré syndrome. *Ann Neurol* 1990;27(suppl 1):S22–S24.

Hughes RAC, Swan AV, van Doorn PA. Intravenous immunoglobulin for Guillain-Barré syndrome (review). *Coc4ane Database of Systematic Reviews* 2014, 9:CD002063.

Rosen BA. Guillain-Barré syndrome. *Pediatrics in Review* 2012;33:164–71.

# 24 Heavy Legs and a Sore Back

You are asked to see a 12-year-old boy in the emergency room who was brought in by his parents because of back pain. The pain is midline, low thoracic, and "sore" in quality. It has been increasing for a week, and at first he and his parents thought that it was from tumbling a little roughly when play-fighting with his younger brother. On further questioning in the emergency department, he feels that, just today, his legs feel "heavy," and it turns out that, uncharacteristically, he has not had a bowel movement or voided his bladder since he awoke this morning. On an initial, cursory examination, he can bear weight but keeps his feet widely planted with knees locked, and tends to hold on to objects— he's not sure if this is to cope with the back pain, or because he is weak. His reflexes are extremely brisk in the ankles and knees, and elsewhere normal.

**What do you do now?**

## TRANSVERSE MYELITIS

In addition to a subjective complaint of back pain, this patient has objective findings of long tract dysfunction that, together, point to the possibility of a lesion in the thoracic spinal cord. The hypothesis that he may have an acquired lesion of the spinal cord evolving over the past week immediately frames this case as a potential neurological emergency, since cord compression is among the possible underlying pathologies. However, before defining this possibility further through a more detailed examination and neuroimaging (MRI with and without contrast) of the thoracic spine, it will be important to address the possibility of a superseding *urologic* emergency: bladder outlet obstruction (i.e., autonomic impairment due to myelopathy).

Therefore, a *focused neurological examination* in this context would include assessment of the hypogastric area for bladder distention (possible need for catheterization), formal strength testing of the limbs, and examination with a sharp or light touch stimulus to see if the patient has a dermatomal (an area of skin that is supplied with the nerve fibers of a single posterior spinal root) or truncal level (sensory loss below the spinal cord level) of sensory deficit. The presence of a dermatomal or truncal level of sensory deficit, if present, could also guide neuroimaging. Since an occult neoplastic lesion should be considered, a careful examination for organomegaly and lymphadenopathy is in order. Similarly, considering the possibility of an inflammatory spinal cord lesion such as transverse myelitis, examination for other stigmata of systemic inflammatory disorders (rash, mucosal lesions) is appropriate.

The patient's bladder proves not to be distended, and, following an IV fluid bolus, he voids normal urine. The MRI shows patchy, noncontiguous, nonenhancing, T2 bright lesions in the midthoracic cord, but no other abnormalities are noted. Based on this finding, you proceed with a spinal tap and find a normal opening pressure and glucose but moderately elevated protein (52 mg/dL) and lymphocytic pleocytosis (23 lymphocytes).

These laboratory results provide definitive evidence that this patient has transverse myelitis. At this point, it is appropriate to hospitalize the patient for observation as well as intravenous corticosteroids. This therapy, while lacking a firm evidence basis, has become a standard response in the setting of transverse myelitis, with the objective to shorten the course of the illness. However, retrospective case series suggest that neither treatment with IV high-dose steroids nor plasmapheresis (as a possible alternative) as immunomodulatory therapies do not affect the risk of permanent deficit or progression to multiple sclerosis. As an example of a "clinically isolated syndrome," among demyelinative disorders of the central nervous system, the diagnosis of transverse myelitis itself evokes consideration of differential diagnostic considerations, each with its own implications for monitoring and prognosis (Table 24.1).

Within a few days, a number of laboratory tests have been sent and returned normal: Lyme titer, B12 level, urine organic acids, ANA, sedimentation rate, cerebrospinal fluid oligoclonal bands, and aquaporin antibody. At this point, the parents inquire further about the diagnosis of transverse myelitis—how and why did their son develop this illness, and what is the prognosis?

If causes of secondary myelitis have been excluded, there is little that can be said about "why" a given individual develops transverse myelitis. Approximately one third of patients make a full recovery. In general, the presence or absence of oligoclonal bands does not in itself allow for a definitive prognosis regarding impending multiple sclerosis. Follow-up should include periodic (yearly for 5 years) head MRI; this can help identify the transition to clinically definite multiple sclerosis so as to proactively monitor for this potential sequela.

Researchers distinguish partial from complete transverse myelitis (Boxes 24.1 and 24.2). One implication of this distinction is that the transition rate to multiple sclerosis is higher in those with the more severe "complete transverse myelitis" (less than 50% at 5 years) compared to those with milder weakness, so-called acute partial transverse myelitis (20% to 30% at 5 years).

Serologic testing for neuromyelitis optica (NMO IgG antibodies), also known as Devic disease, is important to perform, particularly in cases where MRI shows a longitudinally contiguous pattern of signal changes over three segments. Some underlying causes of "secondary myelitis" are outlined in Table 24.1. Criteria for Devic disease (NMO) include the presence of both optic neuritis and myelitis without evidence of disease outside of these loci. There may be either a longitudinally contiguous signal change on spinal cord MRI or pleocytosis (more than 50 white blood cells/mm$^3$).

TABLE 24.1 **Differential Diagnosis of Transverse Myelitis with Supportive MRI Findings**

| Condition | Associated Findings | Prognostic/Therapeutic Considerations |
| --- | --- | --- |
| Devic disease (neuromyelitis optica) | Aquaporin antibody; abnormal optic nerve head on ophthalmoscopy; abnormal visual evoked response; longitudinally contiguous MRI abnormality | Protracted recovery; alternate immunomodulatory therapy (cyclophosphamide; rituximab) |
| Multiple sclerosis | Positive CSF oligoclonal bands; other demyelinative lesions on MRI (follow-up or initial) | Alternate (maintenance) immunomodulatory therapy; protracted course |
| Lyme disease | Positive Lyme titer | Usually a monophasic illness; impact of antibiotics uncertain. |
| Lupus | Positive ANA or other inflammatory markers | Screen for other organ system involvement (kidney, cutaneous); alternate (maintenance) immunomodulatory therapy |
| Other secondary causes of myelitis (Sjögren syndrome, primary antiphospholipid antibody syndrome, sarcoidosis, vasculitides) | Dysimmune markers | Screen for other organ system involvement (kidney, cutaneous); alternate (maintenance) immunomodulatory therapy |
| Cord Ischemia | Usually normal CSF | Consider prothrombotic disorder; monophasic illness, initial improvement followed by slow improvement to fixed deficits |
| B12 deficiency | Mevalonic aciduria, low serum B12 level | Replacement parenteral B12 followed by variable recovery |

> **BOX 24.1 Criteria for Complete Acute Transverse Myelitis**
>
> Moderate or severe symmetrical weakness and autonomic (bladder) dysfunction attributable to the spinal cord
> Symmetrical sensory level
> [CSF or MRI evidence of inflammation within the spinal cord may or may not be present.]

> **BOX 24.2 Proposed Criteria for Acute Partial Transverse Myelitis**
>
> Mild sensory and/or motor dysfunction attributable to the spinal cord, bilateral or unilateral; when severe deficits are present, marked asymmetry is observed
> Sensory signs or symptoms attributable to a sensory level or hemi-level or MRI lesion typical of myelitis
> [CSF or MRI evidence of inflammation within the spinal cord may or may not be present.]

A likely outcome in this case will be complete resolution without recurrence. Some case series suggest a relatively low incidence of either persisting deficits or recurrence with evolution toward multiple sclerosis. As noted above, individuals with a diagnosis of transverse myelitis should have periodic MRI follow-up of both the spine and brain, especially considering the (relatively common, compared to other diagnostic considerations) possibility of multiple sclerosis. The outcome of the disorder is, like many neuroinflammatory conditions that adults also experience, more favorable in children compared to adults.

**KEY POINTS TO REMEMBER**

- Typical onset features back pain, irritability, and gait difficulty.
- Emergent imaging of the spine to assess for cord compression; later brain imaging to assess for multi-focal demyelination.
- Monitor myelopathy patients for voiding dysfunction.

Further Reading

Defresne, P, Meyer L, Tardieu M, et al. Efficacy of high dose steroid therapy in children with severe acute transverse myelitis. *J Neurol Neurosurg Psychiatry* 2001;71:272–4.

Miyazawa R, Ikeuchi Y, Tomomasa T, et al. Determinants of prognosis of acute transverse myelitis in children. *Pediatr Intl 2003*;45:512–6.

Scott TF. Nosology of idiopathic transverse myelitis syndromes. *Acta Neurol Scand* 2007;115:371–6.

# 25  A Sudden Loss of Balance

You are called by a pediatrician who has a 4-year-old girl in his office who awoke from a nap with the inability to walk. The mother states her daughter was fine before the nap and now stumbles and falls when standing. She moves "as though she'd drunk too much alcohol," and her speech seems less clear than usual. She had been playing roughly with her hyperactive 8-year-old brother earlier that day, and the mother is wondering if her child may have sustained a concussion.

The girl had enjoyed good health except for occasional ear infections and upper respiratory infections. Four days ago, she developed a cold with rhinorrhea, coughing, and a low-grade fever. The child had been treated with ibuprofen and was recovering. She had been eating well and had no difficulties with vomiting or diarrhea.

The pediatrician says that the child is afebrile, playful, and alert. The general examination was unremarkable except for mild rhinorrhea. There are no rashes. The chest is clear on auscultation and the abdominal examination normal. No nystagmus is noted, visual fields appear intact, and she has no facial asymmetry. The fundi are difficult to visualize. The child has no difficulty reaching for objects and has no tremor. Reflexes could not be elicited.

When the child is placed in the standing position her feet are more widely placed than usual. When she attempts to walk she is very unsteady and falls either to the right or left. Without help from the mother the child tends to fall after taking a few steps. The pediatrician notes that the child does not appear to be upset by her inability to walk.

The pediatrician is concerned that the child has a concussion, stroke or a cerebellar tumor, and wishes to know if you want to obtain an MRI of the brain.

### What do you do now?

## ACUTE CEREBELLAR ATAXIA

You ask to see the child and confirm the pediatrician's history, asking pointed questions about possible access to household medications that may cause ataxia (tricyclic antidepressants, anxiolytics). You confirm examination findings and manage to get a limited funduscopic examination, turning her ability to fix on her mother's face in low illumination into a game. Funduscopy reveals frequent horizontal saccades that had not been so conspicuous on confrontation, but no papilledema. Although you agree that the child should have an MRI of the brain, you reassure the mother that it is unlikely, especially considering the rapid onset of symptoms, the child has a brain tumor.

With this history and neurological examination, the most likely diagnosis in this child would be acute cerebellar ataxia, also sometimes referred to as "cerebellitis," although often there is no definite evidence of brain inflammation. Acute cerebellar ataxia usually occurs in children between 2 and 7 years of age. The onset is often explosive. As in this case, the child may wake up from a nap with the condition. Ataxia varies from mild unsteadiness while walking to complete inability to walk, and bulbar coordination (speech, swallowing, eye movements) may also be involved. Even when the ataxia is severe, the mental functioning is normal. Despite the difficulty walking, the child, unlike the parents, often appears totally unconcerned about his or her state. While, in principle, the possibility of a cerebellar stroke remains, the absence of a history of a serious blow to the head, with immediate, supervening symptoms, makes concussion extremely improbable.

While the sudden onset of ataxia is concerning, it is likely that the child has a benign condition. Often the first thought is that the child has a posterior fossa tumor, but the history of being fine before a nap and then having pronounced ataxia would be unlikely for a posterior fossa tumor, in which the onset of the ataxia is usually more gradual and headache and vomiting are common. The neurological examination is important. In addition to the ataxia, some children have nystagmus, but this is not a universal finding. Typically in acute cerebellar ataxia the child looks healthy and is not distressed by the condition.

Other conditions that could lead to acute ataxia are listed in Table 25.1. Obtaining a urine toxicology screen would be reasonable in this case. Rare

TABLE 25.1 **Common Causes of Acute Ataxia**

| Cause | Comments |
|---|---|
| Drug ingestion and toxicity | Antihistamines, anticonvulsants, psychotropic medication |
| Brain tumor | Headache, emesis; ataxia has insidious onset |
| Acute cerebellar ataxia | Common, usually postinfectious |
| Miller Fisher syndrome | Associated with ophthalmoplegia and areflexia |
| Cerebellar abscess | Rare, often associated with fever, congenital heart disease, other remote infection |
| Labyrinthitis | Dizziness, vertigo common |
| Head trauma | Ataxia may last days and weeks after head trauma even without loss of consciousness. |
| Opsoclonus-myoclonus syndrome | Usually features myoclonus; paraneoplastic process |
| Cerebellar hemorrhage/ posterior fossa subdural hematoma | Rare, associated with multiple etiologies, may be spontaneous |
| Discitis, acute myelopathy or myelitis | Child may refuse to stand or walks awkwardly due to back pain. |
| Conversion disorder | Rarely occurs in children age <10 years |

causes of acute ataxia include the myoclonus-opsoclonus syndrome and the Miller Fisher syndrome. In the myoclonus-opsoclonus syndrome there are unusual chaotic (multidirectional) eye movements (opsoclonus) in addition to myoclonic jerks of the trunk and extremities and ataxia, although sometimes ataxia precedes myoclonus. Former terms used for the syndrome include dancing eyes and dancing feet syndrome. This condition is a paraneoplastic condition and requires a vigorous search for a neuroblastoma, which may be occult. If deep tendon reflexes cannot be elicited, Guillain-Barré syndrome, or its Miller Fisher variant, should be considered. The

Miller Fisher syndrome is characterized by ataxia, ophthalmoplegia, areflexia, and pupillary abnormalities, without limb weakness.

In acute cerebellar ataxia, a history of a preceding viral illness can usually be elicited. Varicella is a particularly common viral illness occurring before the onset of acute cerebellar ataxia. Other triggering pathogens may include Epstein-Barr, entero-virus, rubeola, parvovirus, and mycoplasma. Sporadic case reports may cloud the more important point that no good epidemiologic evidence supports an association of this condition with vaccinations or with a specific pathogen. Therefore, a laboratory "hunt" for triggers of this benign condition may be of little value to the patient.

Because of the concern about posterior fossa conditions, a head CT or MRI is typically obtained. While the CT is quicker and easier to obtain, the MRI provides better resolution and obviates radiation, whose long-term effects are of increasing concern for children. MRI using FLAIR (fluid attenuation inversion recovery) images will often pick up signal changes in the white matter not only within the cerebellum but also in other white matter areas—evidence of white matter lesions or demyelination on MRI may prompt consideration of Lyme disease in endemic areas, although one must be wary of false-positive serology. A subset of patients with acute disseminated encephalomyelitis (ADEM), which probably has a different pathogenesis than acute cerebellar ataxia without MRI abnormalities, may have primarily cerebellar involvement. Although it is not usually necessary in cases without MRI changes, the spinal fluid examination may show a mild elevation of protein and a few lymphocytes.

Symptoms usually begin to remit after a few days, although a full recovery may take weeks. Most children have a full recovery.

### KEY POINTS TO REMEMBER

- Onset is usually abrupt—over hours to days.
- Ataxia occurs in the context of an otherwise healthy-appearing child.
- Posterior fossa lesions (stroke, demyelination, tumor) must be ruled out.
- Recovery usually occurs but may take months to years.

Further Reading

Desai J, Mitchell WG. Acute cerebellar ataxia, acute cerebellitis, and opsoclonus-myoclonus syndrome. *J Child Neurol* 2012;27:1482-8.

Gieron-Korthals MA, Westberry KR, Emmanuel PJ. Acute childhood ataxia: 10-year experience. *J Child Neurol* 1994;9:381-4.

Gupte G, Stonehouse M, Wassmer E, et al. Acute disseminated encephalomyelitis: a review of 18 cases in childhood. *J Paediatr Child Health* 2003;39:336-42.

Jones CT. Childhood autoimmune neurologic diseases of the central nervous system. *Neurol Clin* 2003;21:745-64.

Maggi G, Varone A, Aliberti F. Acute cerebellar ataxia in children. *Childs Nerv Syst* 1997;13:542-5.

Stonehouse M, Gupte G, Wassmer E, Whitehouse WP. Acute disseminated encephalomyelitis: recognition in the hands of general paediatricians. *Arch Dis Child* 2003;88:122-4.

# 26 Darting Eyes

You are called to the pediatric floor by the pediatric house staff to see an 18-month-old girl who presents with episodes of falling. The mother reports that over the past week the child has been unsteady and falls more than usual. At approximately the same time the girl became shaky and would sometimes drop objects. The mother also is concerned about "funny" eye movements.

The girl is the first child of this 29-year-old woman, who states that the pregnancy, labor, and delivery went well and the child was discharged home with the mother the day after delivery. Development has been normal and other than a few colds the child has been healthy. There is no family history of a neurological disorder.

On examination the girl is noted to be irritable, but is consolable by the mother. The child has some subtle jerks of the arms and legs during your interview and examination. These are multifocal in that they involve both distal and proximal segments of her limbs and shoulder girdle. These movements are of low amplitude, and barely perceptible, but according to the mother they were not present a week ago. On cranial nerve examination you note that her eyes are darting about in a very quick, unpredictable manner. The eyes move together, but the saccadic movements occur in different directions—horizontally, vertically, and diagonally. She can follow a toy for a few seconds, then a saccade interrupts her ocular smooth pursuit. Because of these chaotic eye movements, it is not possible to see the fundi. The remainder of the cranial nerve examination is normal. When reaching for objects there is a tremor in the upper extremities. While strength and sensation, observed through her response to light touch, and her spontaneous movements, appear normal, her reflexes are difficult to elicit. Upon standing there is truncal titubation and the child cannot walk without falling.

The house staff has already obtained an MRI, EEG, electrolytes, CBC, and liver function tests, all of which are normal.

**What do you do now?**

## OPSOCLONUS-MYOCLONUS SYNDROME

When faced with a patient with presumed neurological disease, the first step is to try to determine where the pathology is located. The eye movements you are seeing are referred to as opsoclonus, a condition of uncontrolled eye movements. Opsoclonus consists of rapid, involuntary, multidirectional (horizontal and vertical), unpredictable, conjugate fast eye movements. Opsoclonus is thought to be secondary to abnormalities in the midbrain. The limb movements, being abrupt and nonrhythmic, represent myoclonus. Myoclonus may reflect pathology diffusely, or at several different levels of the central nervous system (e.g., spinal cord, cerebellum, cerebral cortex). The ataxia in this case could point to a cerebellar pathology underlying the myoclonus, although it could also be caused by the child's myoclonus.

The constellation of findings here compels a diagnosis of the opsoclonus-myoclonus syndrome, also called opsoclonus-myoclonus-ataxia, Kinsbourne syndrome, myoclonic encephalopathy of infants, or dancing eyes–dancing feet syndrome. This child has a typical presentation, with both the opsoclonus and myoclonus occurring at the onset—in some cases, weeks of cerebellar ataxia precede the more characteristic signs, thus delaying the diagnosis. As the disorder progresses there is increased severity of the truncal myoclonus, which results in impaired standing and walking. The opsoclonus is usually maximal at the onset of the disorder and then subsides in intensity, and disappears when the child is sleeping. In some children the myoclonus is exacerbated by intention.

The syndrome is associated with neuroblastoma, with the opsoclonus and myoclonus heralding the tumor prior to its diagnosis. This is a paraneoplastic syndrome in which the cancer, precipitating neuroimmune activity, results in neurological dysfunction. Thus the neurological dysfunction is not due to a direct invasion of neural tissue by tumor. The physician must undertake a careful investigation for occult neuroblastoma in all infants and children with the opsoclonus-myoclonus syndrome. An underlying neuroblastoma, present in about 50% of cases, may be quite difficult to detect, prompting extensive scanning of the neck and trunk. Once the tumor is found, removed, and medically treated, symptoms may resolve over months or years (although they may persist indefinitely).

Children without underlying neuroblastoma may in some cases have a history of a prior infection, usually viral. Cerebrospinal fluid may show an elevated protein level and a mild lymphocytic pleocytosis, but this does not distinguish paraneoplastic from para-infectious opsoclonus-myoclonus syndrome. Likewise, serum antineuronal antibodies have in some cases been found in patients with both postinfectious and neuroblastoma-associated opsoclonus-myoclonus syndrome.

Treatment options have included ACTH and corticosteroids (prednisone or methylprednisolone) at high dosages. Intravenous immunoglobulins and immunosuppressive drugs such as cyclophosphamide, azathioprine, and rituximab may be helpful in some cases. The prognosis is quite variable; complete or partial remission may occur and is not dependent on the etiology.

### KEY POINTS TO REMEMBER

- Opsoclonus, a key feature of this disorder, is distinguishable from other forms of nystagmus by conjugate, darting movements in varying directions. The directions of the eye movements are not predictable.
- Ataxia can be secondary to truncal myoclonus or primary cerebellar involvement.
- Investigation for occult neuroblastoma is warranted.
- Steroids or immune modulation therapy can be useful.

Further Reading

Anand G, Bridge H, Rackstraw P, et al. Cerebellar and cortical abnormalities in paediatric opsoclonus-myoclonus syndrome. *Dev Med Child Neurol* 2015;57:265–72.

Connolly AM, Pestronk A, Mehta S, et al. Serum autoantibodies in childhood opsoclonus-myoclonus syndrome: an analysis of antigenic targets in neural tissues. *J Pediatr* 1997;130:878–84.

Desai J, Mitchell WG. Acute cerebellar ataxia, acute cerebellitis, and opsoclonus-myoclonus syndrome. *J Child Neurol* 2012;27:1482–8.

Dyken P, Kolar O. Dancing eyes, dancing feet: infantile polymyoclonia. *Brain* 1968;91:305–20.

Mitchell WG, Snodgrass SR. Opsoclonus-ataxia due to childhood neural crest tumors: a chronic neurologic syndrome. *J Child Neurol* 1990;5:153–8.

Pranzatelli MR, Travelstead AL, Tate ED, et al. B- and T-cell markers in opsoclonus-myoclonus syndrome: immunophenotyping of CSF lymphocytes. *Neurology* 2004;62:1526–32.

Singhi, P. Clinical profile and outcome of children with opsoclonus-myoclonus syndrome. *J Child Neurol* 2014;29:58–61.

Tate ED, Allison TJ, Pranzatelli MR, Verhulst SJ. Neuroepidemiologic trends in 105 U.S. cases of pediatric opsoclonus-myoclonus syndrome. *J Pediatr Oncol Nurs* 2005;22:8–19.

Warrier RP, Kini R, Besser A, Wiatrak B, Raju U. Opsomyoclonus and neuroblastoma. *Clin Pediatr (Phila)* 1985;24:32–4.

# 27  Walking on Tiptoes

The parents of a 6-year-old boy have brought him to your office because of concerns about his gait. There are five other children in the family, and the parents have always noticed that this child's gait was more awkward than his siblings. The family says they were told by their pediatrician that the boy probably had a mild form of cerebral palsy.

In reviewing the history, you learn that the child had a normal birth and had normal early developmental milestones except for a delay in walking. He did not walk until age 18 months and did not run until 36 months. The parents noted that his legs were often stiff, "as though he had Parkinson's disease." He competed poorly in sports where running was required. Despite these problems, the parents felt he had been improving until the past few months, when they observed that he was having worse difficulty with walking and running. He was increasingly walking on his toes and complained of discomfort in his legs. Inquiring about voiding problems, you learn that while he had previously been dry in the morning, recently he has been having nocturnal enuresis.

On examination you find a delightful, bright 6-year-old child who volunteers that he has been having pain in his legs, pointing to his calves. The neurological examination shows normal cranial nerve function. His upper extremities are strong, with symmetrical deep tendon reflexes. Cerebellar function is normal as measured by finger-to-nose and rapid alternating movements. In the lower extremities you find a velocity-dependent increase in tone when you passively flex his knees in supine position, and 3+ reflexes. He has extensor plantar reflexes bilaterally. He walks on his toes and cannot stand on his heels. Sensory examination reveals patchy loss of pinprick sensation on his calves. Position and vibration sensation are normal.

**What do you do now?**

## TETHERED CORD

All the signs and symptoms in this child point to a spinal cord problem. The upper extremities demonstrate normal function, making it difficult to conceive of a lesion in the brain that would account for the neurological findings. Considering the longstanding nature of ostensible myelopathy in this patient, you examine the child's back and discover a dermal sinus in the sacral region surrounded by a small tuft of hair. You probe the sinus with a sterile Q-tip and find it extends approximately 5 mm. You immediately order an MRI of the lumbar spine.

A change in gait associated with leg pain and enuresis requires prompt investigation. For example, although the lack of a sensory level would argue against it, a spinal cord tumor in the lumbar sacral region could account for the findings. But the fact that this child never walked normally suggests that this is a developmental abnormality. The discovery of the dermal sinus adds further support for spinal dysraphism as the basis of this child's problems. Taken together, the history and physical findings make tethered spinal cord most likely.

The spinal cord is said to be "tethered" when it is abnormally attached within the spinal canal. This can occur in spina bifida, when the cord attaches to scar tissue at the time of surgical closure of the spine, or in spina bifida occulta, where an outward defect is not readily apparent. A thickened filum terminale, a lipoma, a dermal sinus, or diastematomyelia (a bifid spinal cord) may anchor the conus medullaris to the base of the vertebrae (Fig. 27–1). Tethered cord also occurs in children with associated anomalies such as caudal regression, or Dandy Walker syndrome.

Dermal sinuses are often marked by a tuft of hair or skin discoloration, due to abnormal invagination of ectoderm into the posterior closure site of the neural tube. As in this case, most sinuses terminate subcutaneously as a blind pouch or dermoid cyst. The cyst may alternatively extend through the bifid spinal vertebra into the dura.

Signs and symptoms of a tethered cord typically feature conspicuous upper motor signs (toe walking, hyperreflexia, spasticity, and lower extremity weakness) but also include changes in bowel control, incomplete emptying of the bladder, urinary tract infections, persistent back pain, increasing scoliosis, decreased sensation in the legs or feet, and stumbling.

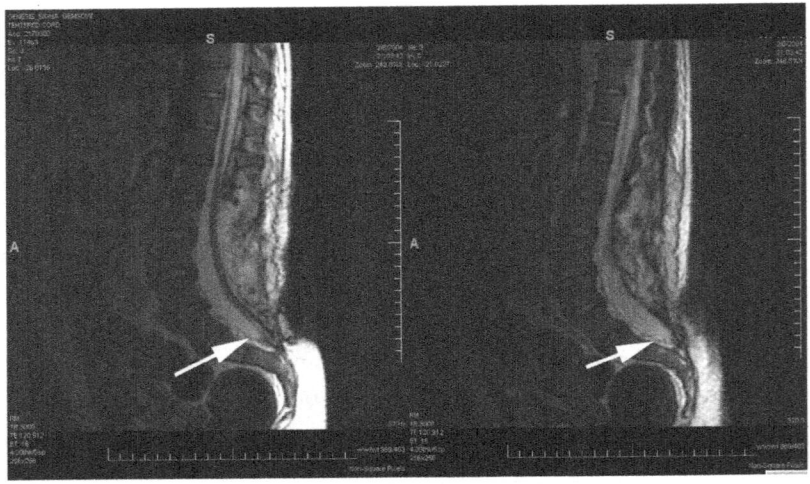

**FIGURE 27-1** MRI of cord tethered to the lower sacral region. The arrow points to the downwardly displaced conus into the sacral region This 4-year-old had lower extremity spasticity and toe walking.

A common presentation is of asymmetric talipes with a small foot, weakness of or wasting of muscles below the knees, loss of ankle jerks, and sensory loss in the leg. The results of the neurological examination vary widely depending on the extent of the tethering and traction effects on the lower cord. Children with relatively milder symptoms of tethered cord, such as clumsy gait or urinary control dysfunction, typically have normal or mildly increased reflexes and extensor plantar responses. Children with more severe deficits have loss of reflexes and foot deformities, and neurogenic voiding difficulties.

The MRI is the appropriate diagnostic test and is very helpful in defining the anatomical abnormalities. Surgical correction of the tethering prevents further deterioration of neurological function and often reverses some of the deficits.

> **KEY POINTS TO REMEMBER**
>
> - A progressive deterioration in gait requires an immediate investigation; cerebral palsy is a static condition and should not lead to increasing neurological impairment.

- Consider a tethered cord in children with deterioration in gait who have a dermal sinus.
- When evaluating the spinal cord for tumors or dysraphism, MRI (with contrast if the suspicion for tumor is strong) is the preferred imaging test.
- Tethering is possible in a patient with a normally positioned cord on MRI ("tight filum"); check for neurological, dermatological, or urological signs.
- Bladder function should be evaluated in all children with known or suspected tethered cord.

Further Reading

Bui CJ, Tubbs RS, Oakes WJ. Tethered cord syndrome in children: a review. *Neurosurg Focus* 2007;23:1–9.

Cornips EMJ, Verelijken IM, Beuls EA, et al. Clinical characteristics and surgical outcome in 25 cases of childhood tight filum syndrome. *Eur J Paediatr Neurol* 2012;16:103–17.

Drake JM. Surgical management of the tethered spinal cord—walking the fine line. *Neurosurg Focus* 2007;23:1–4.

Guerra LA, Pike J, Milks J, Barrowman N, Leonard M. Outcome in patients who underwent tethered cord release for occult spinal dysraphism. *J Urol* 2006;176:1729–32.

Hertzler DA 2nd, DePowell JJ, Stevenson CB, Mangano FT. Tethered cord syndrome: a review of the literature from embryology to adult presentation. *Neurosurg Focus* 2010;29:E1.

Lew SM, Kothbauer KF. Tethered cord syndrome: an updated review. *Pediatr Neurosurg* 2007;43:236–48.

Michelson DJ, Ashwal S. Tethered cord syndrome in childhood: diagnostic features and relationship to congenital anomalies. *Neurol Res* 2004;26:745–53.

Milhorat TH. Association of Chiari malformation type I and tethered cord syndrome: preliminary results of sectioning filum terminale. *Surg Neurol* 2009;72:20–35.

Yamada S. Tethered cord syndrome in adults and children. *Neurol Res* 2004;26:717–8.

Yamada S, Won DJ, Siddiqi J, Yamada SM. Tethered cord syndrome: overview of diagnosis and treatment. *Neurol Res* 2004;26:719–21.

# 28 The Boy Who Kept Rolling His Eyes

You are seeing a 9-year-old boy brought in by his parents because of a concerning array of movements. Four months ago, about 2 weeks after an upper respiratory infection had resolved, he began having sudden, forceful blinking. When asked about the blinking he explained that his eyes felt itchy. Suspecting allergies, his pediatrician recommended an antihistamine, and within a week the eye blinking stopped. Then, 2 weeks later the patient began having eye-rolling movements, sometimes with a brief head tilt. Suspecting possible absence seizures, his family practitioner sent him for consultation. On further questioning, there had been other events occurring without any apparent precipitant the prior summer: sudden head-shaking movements, at varying times of day. Also, his father recalls correcting his son a few months back for making frequent grunting sounds, as though he was rudely clearing his throat, and then the grunting sounds went away. In the kind of sequence that sometimes leads parents to wonder if the doctor will actually believe them, the movements have stopped in the month since the appointment was made.

When asked about the movements, the boy mentions that sometimes other students in his class have made fun of him, although he doesn't say that the movements are bothering him. He seems defensive, perhaps because he has been corrected, but also does not remember the head-shaking or the eye-rolling movements. It was precisely this lack of recollection on the part of the patient that led his physician to refer with consideration of absence seizures. The patient states that he could sometimes feel the forceful blinking movements "coming on," and could actually stop the blinking, at least for a while. Most of the time, however, he didn't notice any of the movements as much as other people did.

Medical history reveals that there had been an evaluation for attention-deficit/hyperactivity disorder (ADHD). His physician had then recommended a stimulant medication, but it made him anxious and aggressive, and was discontinued. Moreover, his parents had differed on the significance of the patient's ADHD signs and symptoms and their treatment, so the whole question was put aside. This family asks where these movements came from, why do they seem to start and stop when they do, and what do they mean about their son's future?

**What do you do now?**

## TIC DISORDERS

About 10% of children—especially boys—have tics, usually for just a few months or years. Tics are extremely common in 7- to 12-year-old children. Key features that identify these movements as tics include that they (1) involve anatomical regions at the level of the shoulder girdle and above (although there are exceptions); (2) are arhythmic in their repetitiveness, although stereotyped; (3) wax and wane in the course of a day, and over weeks, with one movement pattern replacing or overlapping with another; and (4) at least in some cases have a premonitory cognitive component. Three tic syndromes are chronic motor tic, chronic vocal and motor tic (i.e., Tourette syndrome), and transient tic, with the latter type being the most common.

The vast majority of tic disorders are fundamentally benign and genetically based. In rare cases they may stem from an underlying tumor, encephalitis, or degenerative syndrome (Huntington disease), and there are some children whose tics occur only in the context of stimulant therapy for ADHD. PANDAS (pediatric autoimmune disorders associated with streptococcal infection) remains controversial as an underlying cause of tics of abrupt onset with personality changes (rigidity, irritability, obsessiveness) and occurs rarely, if at all, in our experience.

As in most cases, this patient's tics are not a symptom of some underlying disease. Often the larger concerns for the patient have to do with comorbidities, especially attention deficit. Although tics themselves are not the cause of distractibility or inattention, tic disorders are often associated with attention problems. Medication is rarely recommended—only if the tics get very intense and bother the child. The key is educating others around the child to ignore the tics, so that the tics don't end up bothering the child just because they bother others. A different ADHD medicine might be helpful, but meta-analyses indicate that the onset of tics in association with stimulants is probably most often a chance association. These medicines may be used and do not characteristically worsen tics.

Obsessive-compulsive disorder (OCD) represents another comorbidity often associated with tics—after all, the French term for tics has historically been *tic compulsif* (although tics in themselves are *not* considered a manifestation of OCD). Here it is important to remember that obsessive-compulsive trait is probably much more common than OCD; the difference relates to whether or not there is in fact a significant and frequent functional impact related to obsessive behaviors or compulsive thoughts (DSM-5).

Often the question arises as to whether motor tics represent a harbinger of impending Tourette syndrome. While this is certainly a possibility, most tics arising in children ultimately play out as a *transient motor tic* disorder and do not persist into late adolescence or adulthood. In the setting of Tourette syndrome (defined by the presence of persistent vocal *and* motor tics for a year), tics also often recede in the latter part of the second decade of life, while symptoms related to comorbid obsessive disorder may intensify into young adulthood, especially among those with higher IQ.

Sometimes what seems most surprising about tics is the level of concern they provoke. Once the diagnosis of tics is established, as it can almost always be, by history and physical examination alone, laboratory tests are generally not helpful. But the question arises whether a medicine is needed, or what else can be done to stop the tics. Since the most common ill effect of tics for the person who has them usually relates to social stigma or misunderstanding, the most important intervention is this setting is usually educational. Reframing the tics may include (1) realizing how common they are; (2) recognizing that unwanted attention evoked by tics can represent a "teaching" moment for the child with tics; (3) reviewing the varied natural course of tics; and (4) discussing the real possibility that there are functional advantages that are probably associated with tics (e.g., quicker reflexes).

---

**KEY POINTS TO REMEMBER**

- The temporal course may be transient (months) or chronic (years).
- Tourette syndrome is distinguished by the presence of chronic motor and vocal (audible) tics.
- Pharmacotherapy is usually not necessary.
- Usually no laboratory testing is necessary.
- Comorbidities, especially ADHD, may be of more consequence to the child.

Further Reading

Bloch MH, Peterson BS, Scahill L, et al. Adulthood outcome of tic and obsessive-compulsive symptom severity in children with Tourette syndrome. *Arch Pediatr Adolesc Med* 2006;147:65–9.

Cohen SC, Mulqueen JM, Ferracioli-Oda E, et al. Meta-analysis: risk of tics associated with psychostimulant use in randomized, placebo-controlled trials. *J Am Acad Child Adolesc Psychiatry* 2015;54:728–36.

Jeon S, Walkup JT, Woods DW, et al. Detecting a clinically meaningful change in tic severity in Tourette syndrome: A comparison of three methods. *Contemp Clin Trials* 2013;36:414–20.

Oakley C, Mahone EM, Morris-Berry C, et al. Primary complex motor stereotypies in older children and adolescents: clinical features and longitudinal follow-up. *Pediatr Neurol* 2015;52:398–403.

Shaw ZA, Coffey BJ. Tics and Tourette syndrome. *Pediatr Clin North Am* 2014;37:269–86.

# 29  A Sudden Collapse

A family medicine nurse practitioner has referred a 14-year-old girl to the ER because of a change in gait, and you are called by the ER physician to consult there. You arrive to the ER examination room to find the patient sitting supported with her parents in attendance. She states that her legs suddenly "gave out" while she was getting out of the car when her mother was dropping her off at a friend's house just 2 hours before, and that she didn't trust herself to stand independently since then. Her mother reports that she seemed to abruptly collapse, grasping for the open car door and partly holding herself up, until her mother could come around and help ease her back in to the rear car seat. There were no sensory or voiding concerns or complaints.

    Medical history is remarkable only for a mild concussion sustained on the basketball court about 1 year earlier when another player's elbow struck her head. This mild concussion manifested as some dizziness for a day, and persistent, migraine-like headache for 5 weeks. The patient is said to be of an anxious disposition.

Examination shows normal cranial nerves and strength in her arms, and normal reflexes, but she is unable to raise her legs singly from a supine position. When assisted to a standing position, she crouches, holding on to the examiner on one side and her parent on the other, abruptly shifting her weight from one leg to another, as though catching herself to prevent a fall.

### What do you do now?

## CONVERSION DISORDER

The striking inconsistency in this patient's motor examination is demonstrated in the contrast between formal testing of the iliopsoas muscle group (fails to perform an active leg raise—apparently no better than 2 out of 5 strength for supine leg raise using the standard power assessment scale) and the relatively good function in the same muscle group when a different functional test is used. Her crouched, shifting position indicates at least 4+ strength in the hip flexors/extensors in the "standing" challenge. This inconsistency strongly suggests that the patient is suffering from a so-called functional neurological symptom disorder (formerly conversion disorder or psychogenic movement disorder [now archaic]). Although the point has been made that the diagnosis of a functional neurological symptom disorder should be made only when alternative possible causes of the patient's symptoms have been rigorously excluded (i.e., "diagnosis of exclusion"), others have made a strong case that the pattern of signs and symptoms in these disorders is so characteristic that this diagnosis can be made inductively.

Functional neurological symptom disorders have a history, traveling under one nosologic system or another, as long as that of neurology itself. While psychological and behavioral features, such as anxious personality type or an indifferent or vague character in how the history of symptoms is disclosed, are common in functional neurological disorder, such features are more incidental than they are foundational to the diagnosis. It should be noted that, whether because they are unknown to the patient and family or because they are not pertinent, many cases of functional neurological disorder do not, at least initially, feature a prior or ongoing psychosocial stressor. In the present case, one might wonder why the functional gait changes just at the moment that the patient is going to do something enjoyable (i.e., visit a close friend). Just as the point is often made that there is often no ostensible psychosocial stressor elicited from patients with functional neurological disorder (or from their families), it is also true that their symptoms, when paroxysmal or undulating, may often worsen even at comfortable or happy moments of their lives. If nothing else, such paradoxical patterns offer a lesson in the sometimes inscrutable nature of the subconscious mind.

The key to diagnosis is that the signs and symptoms, while they may suggest a neurological problem, are essentially incompatible with any known neurological condition. In the present case, the wide variation in this patient's apparent leg strength spanning minutes of observation strongly suggests that her weakness is related either to poor effort (e.g., feigning) or subconscious factors (e.g., functional neurological disorder). Incidentally, it is very improbable that complications of the prior concussion (e.g., epilepsy, arachnoid cyst, dural arteriovenous malformation, chronic subdural hematoma) account for the current symptoms.

One caveat to the preceding statement stems from the diagnostic problem of "functional overlay." Could the patient, despite the probable psychosomatic basis of the signs and symptoms, have an underlying neurological problem onto which the more conspicuous findings have been overlain? Such a consideration sometimes compels, at least at the first visit, a more conservative diagnostic stance, such as the rubric "medically unexplained symptoms." The possibility that some patients with functional neurological disorders may *also* have an underlying neurological condition undoubtedly drives much laboratory testing in these cases.

Considering the association of conversion disorder in teenaged girls with prior abuse, you perform a confidential interview and learn that she currently feels "safe" with the peers and adults in her life, and that she has always felt safe in the past. After observation in the ER for 2 hours, the patient is feeling stronger and seems to be walking without difficulty. After lengthy discussion, including mention of the associated stigma, with patient and family regarding the diagnosis of Functional Neurological Disorder, she is discharged from the ER with plans for close follow-up—once with the neurologist, thereafter with her primary care practitioner.

Functional neurological disorders comprise motor deficits (tremor, paralysis, dyskinesia), sensory deficits (numbness), and seizure-like episodes. A growing fMRI literature is beginning to identify the pathology in these diverse disorders as a problem of network "miswiring." New patients to neurologists include many patients with no apparent underlying neuropathology to be identified, many of whom, in turn, prove to have some variant of a functional neurological symptom disorder. Misunderstandings, and compounding of stigma, commonly arise when the clinician presumes that the patient is at some level feigning, as in factitious disorder, or malingering. In fact, feigning seems to be relatively rare compared to the disorders of executive functioning that underlie functional neurological symptom disorders.

Teamwork is essential, with a firm collaborative approach among neurologist, psychologist, generalist, and, in some cases, psychiatrist (there is not a strong evidence base to support pharmacotherapy in this setting). Many patients with functional neurological disorders do well and benefit from follow-up visits. Such follow-up not only can provide emotional support to the patient and family but will inevitably make better prognosticators of us!

---

**KEY POINTS TO REMEMBER**

- Adolescents tend to present with either seizure-like spells, movement disorders (tremor), sensory deficit (visual impairment, numbness), or weakness.
- Psychodynamic mechanisms or stressors are often not apparent.
- These patients call for multidisciplinary, coordinated care, and explicit discussion of credibility concerns and stigma.
- While some "rule-out" laboratory testing may be required (especially EEG for seizures), the diagnosis may be apparent from history and physical examination.

---

Further Reading

Nicholson TR, Stone J, Kanaan RA. Conversion disorder—a problematic diagnosis. *J Neurol Neurosurg Psychiatry* 2011;82:1267–73.

Allin M, Streeruwitz A, Curtis V. Progress in understanding conversion disorder. *Neuropsychiatric Dis Treatment* 2005;1:205–9.

# 30 The Headache That Wouldn't Go Away

A 14-year-old girl is referred because of headaches that started 2 years ago. Initially, back in seventh grade, she had "normal" headaches a few times a month, although at least twice she had to miss school because of a bad headache. Then, in December of her eighth-grade year, there was an incident playing basketball in gym where another player "accidentally" shoved her, and she struck her occiput upon falling to the wooden floor. She felt dizzy and lightheaded for the rest of that day and had a very bad generalized headache that persisted for almost 2 months. For the next 4 months, she started to experience bad frontal headaches associated with sensitivity to loud sounds and bright light almost weekly.

    Although the headaches were better over the summer, this year, in ninth grade, she has noticed the headaches increasing in frequency. Now, in January of ninth grade, she rarely has a headache-free day. She experiences some nausea, but no vomiting, on days when the headache is at its worse, but she does not identify a circadian pattern to the headache (i.e., time of day when it is worse). Although it is hard to tell if it is helpful, she takes a nonsteroidal anti-inflammatory medicine almost every day, sometimes twice a day.

Her general and neurological examination are mostly normal, including normal jaw excursions and absence of sinus or other point tenderness. However, she is significantly overweight, with a body mass index of 32, and she does have a mild limitation in range of horizontal head movements, with some tightness of the bilateral trapezius muscles. On funduscopic exam, you can make out the presence of venous pulsations when you look at the veins radiating from the disc center of her right eye.

**What do you do now?**

## CHRONIC DAILY HEADACHE/MIGRAINE

Headache is not only one of the most common complaints that generalists hear from their patients, but it is also a concern with one of the broadest differential diagnostic considerations of any single complaint. The possibilities include a wide range of metabolic, inflammatory, infectious, neoplastic, iatrogenic, toxic, circulatory, and endocrinological causes. The consideration that primary headache disorders appear far more commonly than do secondary headaches means that generalists and specialists alike must be constantly on guard against possible "availability bias" setting up the potential for a missed diagnosis of a headache with an underlying cause.

So what are some possible causes of secondary headache in the present situation? Being overweight, this patient is at risk for sleep apnea, and it will be important to check in about snoring or excessive daytime sleepiness. Idiopathic intracranial hypertension (IIH), formerly known as pseudotumor syndrome, can present with chronic headache as a sole complaint and finding, and is also more common in overweight persons, though the funduscopic examination weighs against this possibility. It should be noted, too, that obesity is also a risk factor for so-called chronification or progression of migraine from episodic to chronic temporal pattern of headache. While it is unclear whether weight loss in this setting may improve headache, such a goal is sensible in principle considering the many health issues associated with obesity.

Although it sometimes presents without papilledema (IIHWOP), the presence of venous pulsations, which is strongly (although not infallibly) indicative of normal intracranial pressure, can here reassure us against idiopathic intracranial hypertension. The same consideration applies to the possibility of hydrocephalus, chronic subdural hematoma, chronic meningitis, or sinovenous thrombosis. If one of these were the cause of headache, one would expect other signs and symptoms, and more definitive related signs of intracranial hypertension.

Of these, sinovenous thrombosis, IIH, and chronic meningitis appear to be the most common "lookalikes" to chronic daily headache. Accordingly, there may be an interest in sequential head MRI followed by spinal tap with opening pressure to address these possibilities. Finally, in various regions of the United States (e.g., Northeast, Pacific Northwest), the spirochetal infection known as Lyme disease may present as a chronic headache due to chronic meningitis, although the winter season presentation here would be less typical.

The prevalence of chronic daily headache as a type of primary headache syndrome is extremely high—near 5% of the population within this age group by some estimates. Therefore, in this setting, the clinician needs to be alert for comorbid, rather than underlying, conditions. The first consideration of a diagnosis comorbid to primary, chronic daily headache is depression or anxiety. Aside from being frequent in the general population, affective disorders may run as high as 30% to 40% among teenagers with chronic daily headache. Second, substance abuse may contribute to chronic daily headache, especially to the extent that it may interfere with sleep patterns or add to stress. A confidential, one-on-one interview should be performed to check in about this possibility. The third is medication overuse—it will be important to encourage the patient to desist from her frequent consumption of NSAIDs, since her headache may be exacerbated, or caused, by this pattern. Finally, the incidence of obesity, possibly with an associated sleep disorder, probably is increased among patients with chronic daily headache. As noted above, it is not entirely clear that weight loss would improve the headache, the patient should be advised of this association, and be provided some resources and counseling toward the goal of weight loss.

In this case, historical characteristics of the chronic daily headache—that is, association with light and sound sensitivity—identify it as chronic migraine. While she may have had a few migraine headaches before the basketball incident, the mild concussion that she sustained has apparently precipitated a definitive pattern of migraine headache during the months after the blow. Since her headaches during the last months of ninth grade were intermittent, she probably did not have a postconcussive headache syndrome per se, but rather migraine triggered by trauma.

Therapeutic considerations for chronic migraine can be divided into nonpharmacological lifestyle factors that have to do with daily behavior patterns and pharmacological approaches. Relevant lifestyle factors include stress management/coping styles, sleep pattern, the content of her diet (especially caffeine or theobromine [in chocolate] consumption), and exercise. Preventive pharmacological approaches show variable success and include tricyclic antidepressants, topiramate, valproate (with caution, considering side effects including teratogenicity). Serotonin–norepinephrine reuptake inhibitors (SNRIs) may be helpful in the setting of associated anxiety or depression. Some centers start with supplements or vitamins that have shown success in combatting episodic migraine (e.g., vitamin B2/riboflavin, magnesium, vitamin D).

> **KEY POINTS TO REMEMBER**
> - Even relentless and disabling headaches can be "primary" (i.e., without a single underlying cause) in nature.
> - History may reveal that a chronic daily headache in fact represents a variant of migraine.
> - Chronic daily headache with normal examination findings evokes a differential diagnosis including depression, chronic meningitis, sinovenous thrombosis, and idiopathic intracranial hypertension.
> - A combination of lifestyle and pharmacotherapeutic interventions can be helpful for patients with primary chronic daily headaches.

Further Reading

Bigal ME, Rapoport AM. Obesity and chronic daily headache. *Curr Pain Headache Rep* 2012;16:101–9.

Cho SJ, Chu MK. Risk factors of chronic daily headache or chronic migraine. *Curr Pain Headache Rep* 2015;19:465.

# 31 Headache: To Scan, or Not to Scan?

An 11-year-old boy is referred for headache and an MRI abnormality. He says that, as a current fifth grader, he doesn't think he had headaches until third grade. Overall, the headaches started intermittently and were mild and felt in a generalized way throughout his head. However, through the fall of fifth grade, the headaches have become more severe and more common. Also, now the headaches are especially frontal or bitemporal, although not lateralized, and they are not associated with other signs or symptoms that might support a diagnosis of migraine (no light or sound sensitivity, inconsistent stomach upset without vomiting, headache is nonthrobbing and not exercise induced).

During the 2-month wait leading up to your appointment with him, his parents had brought him to the nurse practitioner/primary care clinician frequently, and, fearful for their son, pleaded for a neuroimaging study. While the nurse practitioner was not entirely sure this was appropriate, he went ahead and ordered a head MRI without contrast a month before your appointment with him. This study was entirely normal, except for what the radiologist called "cerebellar tonsillar herniation through the foramen magnum, 6 mm, probable Chiari I malformation."

**What do you do now?**

## CHIARI I MALFORMATION

You examine the boy and find that his general and neurological examination all seem to be normal. Next, you review the head MRI and confirm the Chiari I finding. The parents, knowing of this finding from their primary care clinician, are most anxious to know next steps.

Of all the incidental findings that may arise when studies such as head MRIs are used as "screening" tools, Chiari I malformation is perhaps the most troublesome, because it is clear that there are some individuals in whom this finding underlies headache, among other signs and symptoms. Evidence-based guidelines that could be used to resolve the question as to whether the finding is significant in any given case have yet to be written, and there is undoubtedly a panoply of "local traditions," algorithms guiding responses to situations such as the one outlined above. A central question here is how to avoid "overdoing," versus inappropriately deferring, a neurosurgical referral for consideration of suboccipital craniectomy. In this case (as in most instances!), a coherent, teamwork approach to the problem among neurosurgeon, generalist, and pediatric neurologist will obviously serve the interests of the patient and his family.

It should be noted that the term "malformation," in the sense of a congenital anomaly, is probably a misnomer, since the lesion more probably represents a deformation following imbalanced hydrostatic pressures across the foramen magnum. Relevant here is the consideration that the prevalence of Chiari I malformation, whether or not it is considered incidental, increases with age. Similar hydrostatic forces likely play a role in the genesis of Chiari II, which *is* present from birth, in association with spinal dysraphism. The presence of other signs and symptoms pertinent, and relatively specific to, Chiari I malformation (Boxes 31.1 to 31.3), would support the case for neurosurgical referral. Of these, the most compelling laboratory finding will probably be the presence of syrinx in the cervical cord. Therefore, if Chiari I malformation is identified, strong consideration should be given to reflexively imaging the cervical cord to identify an associated syringomyelia.

Surgery should in particular be considered in those patients with a known, enlarging syringomyelia, those with refractory occipital headaches, or those with the other objective motor or sensory signs or symptoms

> **BOX 31.1 Historical Findings Indicating Potentially Symptomatic Chiari I Malformation**
>
> Consistent occipital headache location
> Symptoms with neck extension
> New gait difficulty or imbalance
> New voiding difficulty (upper motor neuron)
> Shawl or distal upper extremity sensory disturbance (syrinx, tethered cord?)

> **BOX 31.2 Physical Examination Findings Indicating Potentially Symptomatic Chiari I Malformation**
>
> C2 dermatomal sensory loss
> Downbeat nystagmus
> Limb weakness
> Hyperreflexia, clonus, ataxia
> Upper extremity/shoulder sensory deficit

> **BOX 31.3 Radiological Findings Indicating Potentially Symptomatic Chiari I Malformation**
>
> Cervical syrinx (especially if expanding on serial studies)
> Tethered cord (lumbar MRI)
> Signal change within the cerebellar tonsil parenchyma
> Slowed or blocked flow on dedicated flow studies

outlined in Boxes 31.1 through 31.3. In retrospective series, surgery appears to have a high success rate (75% or greater) in improving headache and syrinx. Syrinx may sometimes be a factor underlying progressive scoliosis; however, it has been pointed out that the mere presence of Chiari I in association with scoliosis, without associated syrinx, could be a noncausal association. The history in the present case should focus on alternate causes of chronic progressive headache that may obviate consideration of the Chiari I malformation as a cause; some possibilities here are outlined in Table 31.1.

When other historical, physical examination, or neuroradiological findings indicative of symptomatic Chiari I are absent, the threshold for neurosurgical referral will likely depend on rapport with the patient and family and the specialist's level of comfort. Of course, the occurrence of

TABLE 31.1  **Historical Features of Some Alternative Causes of Chronic Progressive Headache**

| Historical Clue | Supporting Evidence | Diagnostic Consideration(s) | Implication for Treatment |
| --- | --- | --- | --- |
| Consuming nonprescription or narcotic analgesics | Weak or partial response; consumption ≥4×/week; improvement following restriction | Medication overuse headache | Restrict analgesics |
| Orthostatic intolerance, orthostatic headache, preceding illness or concussion | Orthostatic pulse rise >30 bpm without blood pressure change | Postural orthostatic tachycardia syndrome with associated headache | Fluids, exercise, ?beta blockade |
| Sleep disturbance | Daytime sleepiness, heavy snoring, subjective insomnia | Obstructive sleep apnea or other causes of sleep disturbance | Identify and address contributing factors (e.g., obesity, poor sleep hygiene, stress, medications) |
| Unremitting headache, transient visual disturbance | Papilledema on examination, other neurological findings | Intracranial hypertension (idiopathic, structural) | Spinal tap to reduce intracranial pressure, acetazolamide |
| Low mood, personality change | Psychosocial stressors, vegetative symptoms | Anxiety/depression comorbid to or underlying headache | Pharmacotherapy or counseling for affective disorder |

headache remission following suboccipital craniectomy in some of these cases does not in itself prove that the headache was due to the tonsillar herniation. Some centers use cerebrospinal fluid flow studies to help sort out this question (i.e., inferring that a blockage, or slowing, of flow increases the likelihood that the herniation is symptomatic). The decision regarding neurosurgical referral will depend on the sense of teamwork, coherence, and trust among specialists. When alternative causes of headache appear unlikely (see Table 31.1), neurosurgical referral will often be appropriate even in the absence of other signs and symptoms of symptomatic Chiari I (see Boxes 31.1 through 31.3).

> **KEY POINTS TO REMEMBER**
> - Although this is most commonly an incidental finding, prominent occipital headache may be attributable to Chiari I.
> - Signs and symptoms of Chiari I are varied and include voiding dysfunction, gait difficulty, vertical nystagmus, and upper limb and trunk sensory disturbance.
> - Consider MRI of the cervical spine to assess for associated syringomyelia.
> - Multidisciplinary, coordinated care between generalist, neurologist, and neurosurgeon is needed.
> - Effective treatment of a primary headache can obviously clarify concerns over whether headache is caused by Chiari I.

Further Reading

Arnautovic A, Splavski B, Boop FA, Arnautovic KI. Pediatric and adult Chiari malformation type I surgical series 1965–2013: a review of demographics, operative treatment, and outcomes. *J Neurosurg Pediatr* 2015;15:161–77.

Lee S, Wang K, Cheon J, Phi J, et al. Surgical outcome of Chiari I malformation in children: clinico-radiological factors and technical aspects. *Childs Nervous System* 2014;30:613–23.

McVige JW, Leonardo J. Neuroimaging and the clinical manifestations of Chiari malformation type I. *Curr Pain Headache Rep* 2015;19:18.

Strahle A, Smith BW, Martinez M, et al. The association between Chiari malformation type I, spinal syrinx, and scoliosis. *J Neurosurg Pediatr* 2015;15:607–11.

# Index

Page numbers followed by *f* or *t* indicate a figure or table on the designated page

Absence seizures, 4–7
   EEG signature, 5*f*, 6*f*, 56*f*, 57*f*
   in JME, 55
   treatment, 6
Achondroplasia, 128*t*
Aciduria, 108*t*, 128*t*
Acquired multifocal, T2 bright lesions of the brain, 144*t*
Acromegalic facial features, 95
Acute cerebellar ataxia. *See* ataxia, acute cerebellar
Acute disseminated encephalomyelitis (ADEM), 143, 163
Acute polyneuritis. *See* Guillain-Barré syndrome
Adrenocorticotropic hormone (ACTH) for infantile spasms, 49
Alexander disease, 128*t*
Alternating hemiplegia. *See* hemiplegia, alternating
Alternating hemiplegia of childhood, 11–12
Aminoacidopathies, 108*t*
Amino acid supplementation, 110
Anoxic reflexive epilepsy, 29
Antiepileptic drug therapy
   for benign neonatal sleep myoclonus, 18*t*
   for benign rolandic epilepsy, 24
   for juvenile myoclonic epilepsy, 58
   for Panayiotopoulos syndrome, 35
   for Rett syndrome, 117
   for status epilepticus, 63*t*
Areflexia, 11, 150
Arthrogryposis, 75, 76, 77, 79, 122
Arthrogryposis multiplex congenita, 77
Ataxia, acute cerebellar, 161–63
   causes, 162*t*

Ataxia-telangiectasia, 84*t*
Attention-deficit/hyperactivity disorder (ADHD)
   in fragile-X syndrome, 95
   in neurofibromatosis, 102
   *vs.* absence seizures, 4, 5
Autism spectrum disorder, 5, 95
Autoimmune (transplacentally transmitted antibody) myasthenia gravis, 121
Autonomic seizure, 35
Autosomal dominant inheritance, 70
Autosomal dominant megalencephaly, 129*t*
Autosomal recessive muscular dystrophy, 90*t*
Azathioprine, 168

Becker muscular dystrophy, 89–90, 90*t*
Benign epilepsy of childhood with occipital paroxysms (BECOP), 35
Benign epilepsy with centrotemporal spikes (BECTS), 23–25, 35
   EEG, 24*f*
Benign neonatal sleep myoclonus, 17–18, 18*t*
Benign rolandic epilepsy (BRE). *See* benign epilepsy with centrotemporal spikes (BECTS)
Benzodiazepines, 62
   for alternating hemiplegia, 11
   for status epilepticus, 63
*Borrelia burgdorferi*, 151
Breath-holding spells, 29–31, 30*t*, 116
Buccal midazolam, 12

Café-au-lait spots, 100, 101*f*
*Campylobacter jejuni*, 150
Canavan disease, 128*t*

Carbamazepine, 24, 63
Caudal regression, 173
Central core disease, 77
Cerebellar ataxia, areflexia, pes cavus, optic atrophy and sensorineural hearing loss (CAPOS), 11
Cerebellar hemorrhage/posterior fossa subdural hematoma, 162*t*
Cerebral dysgenesis, 108*t*
Cerebral ischemia (strokes), 135
Cerebral palsy, 81, 83, 85, 87, 89, 174
Charcot Marie Tooth (CMT) disorders, 70–72, 71*t*
Childhood epilepsy, 35
Chronic daily headache, 191–93
Clonazepam, 10, 55, 58
Clonic seizures, 17, 18*t*, 30*t*, 35, 55, 135
Clonic-tonic-clonic seizures, 55
Communicating hydrocephalus, 129*f*
Conduct disorders, 95
Congenital (genetically based) myasthenia gravis, 121
Congenital fiber-type disproportion myopathy, 77
Congenital muscular dystrophies, 77
Congenital muscular dystrophy, 90*t*
Congenital myotonic dystrophy, 77, 78*f*, 79
Congenital X-linked hydrocephalus, with adducted thumbs, 130
Connexin 32 mutation, 72
Conversion disorder, 162*t*, 185–88
Corticoid therapy, 144
Craniofacial dysmorphism, 95
Craniosynostoses, 130
Cyclophosphamide, 156*t*, 168

Dancing eyes-dancing feet syndrome. *See* opsoclonus-myoclonus syndrome
Dandy Walker syndrome, 173
Daydreaming, 4–6, 7*t*
Daytime seizure, 24, 25
Degenerative syndrome (Huntington Disease), 179

Device disease (neuromyelitis optica), 156*t*
Diastematomyelia, 173
Diazepam
  for Panayiotopoulos syndrome, 36
  for seizures, 42, 61
  for status epilepticus, 62, 63*t*
Diffuse hypertonia, 10
Discitis, acute myelopathy of myelitis, 162*t*
Diurnal partial seizures, 23, 24
Dopamine-responsive dystonia, 83–86
  episodic dystonia in children, differential diagnosis, 84*t*
Down syndrome, 137
Duchenne muscular dystrophy, 88–91, 90*t*
Dysdiadochokinesia, 98
Dysmorphologic syndromes, 130
Dystonia/parkinsonism, rapid-onset, 11

Emery-Dreifuss muscular dystrophy, 90*t*
Encephalitis, 179
Encephalopathy
  hyperammonemic, due to urea cycle disorders, 110
  hypoxic-ischemic, 64
  NMDA receptor AB, 143–45, 144*t*
Epidermal nevus syndrome, 128*t*
Epilepsy
  anoxic reflexive epilepsy, 29
  benign epilepsy with centrotemporal spikes, 23–25, 35
  in boys with fragile-X syndrome, 95
  idiopathic generalized epilepsies, 57
  juvenile myoclonic epilepsy, 55–58, 56*f*–57*f*
  status epilepticus, 62–64
  *vs.* alternating hemiplegia of childhood, 11
Episodic ataxia, 11
Ethosuximide, 6
Exercise-induced dystonia, 84*t*
Extrinsic hydrocephalus, 130
Eye jerking, 10

Facial diplegia, 75, 77, 79, 90t, 122
Facioscapulohumeral dystrophy, 90t
Familial neuropathy and associated mutations, 71t
Febrile seizures, 41–42
Floppiness, 11, 119
Flunarizine, 12
Focal seizures, 4–7, 23, 41, 144
Fosphenytoin, 62, 63t
Fragile-X syndrome, 95–96
Fukuyama congenital muscular dystrophy, 90t
Functional neurological disorders, 185–87

Gangliosidosis, 128t
Glutaric aciduria, 128t
Guillain- Barré syndrome (GBS), 149–51, 162
  causes, 149t

Headache
  chronic daily, 191–93
  migraine/migraine-like, 36, 135, 191–93
Head trauma, 162t
Hemiplegia, alternating, 11–12, 84t, 135
Hereditary motor sensory neuropathies. *See* Charcot Marie Tooth (CMT) disorders
Hereditary progressive dystonia with diurnal variation (Segawa disease), 83, 85
Hippocampal stenosis, 42
Huntington disease, 179
Hydrocephalus, 126–30
  accompanying Chiari malformation, 130
  communicating hydrocephalus, 129f
  obstructive hydrocephalus, 128t
  unilateral left hemisphere hydrocephalus due to obstruction of the foramen of Monro, 130f
  *vs.* megalencephaly, 130
Hyperammonemic encephalopathy due to urea cycle disorders, 110

Hyperreflexia, 173
Hypocalcemia, 108t
Hypoglycemia, 108t
Hypomelanosis of Ito, 128t
Hyporeflexia, 70, 79, 149, 150
Hypotonia, 11, 77, 79, 89, 90t, 114, 115, 121, 122, 128t
Hypoventilation, 62
Hypoxia-ischemia, 108t
Hypoxic-ischemic encephalopathy, 64

Idiopathic generalized epilepsy, 57
Idiopathic intracranial hypertension (IIH), 191
  without papilledema (IIHWOP), 191
Immunoglobulins, 168
Immunosuppressive drugs, 168
Incontinentia pigmenti, 128t
Infantile botulism, 121
Infantile spasms, 48–50
  EEG, 49f
  MRI, 50f
Intraventricular hemorrhage, 108t
Intrinsic hydrocephalus, 130
Iris hamartomas (Lisch nodules), 101
Iron deficiency anemia, 30

Juvenile myoclonic epilepsy (JME), 55–58, 55f–57f

Kinsbourne syndrome. *See* opsoclonus-myoclonus syndrome
Krabbe disease, 128t

Labyrinthitis, 162t
Lamotrigine
  for absence seizures, 6
  for juvenile myoclonic epilepsy, 58
  for partial seizures, 24
Late-onset Gastaut Panayiotopoulos syndrome, 35–36
Late-onset neonatal encephalopathy with seizures, 107

Lennox-Gastaut syndrome, 55, 57f
Levetiracetam
   for juvenile myoclonic epilepsy, 57
   for Panayiotopoulos syndrome, 36
   for partial seizures, 24
   for status epilepticus, 63t
Levodopa/carbidopa, 83
Limb-girdle muscular dystrophy, 90t
Liver transplant, 110
Long QT syndrome, 30
Lorazepam, 62, 63t
Lupus CN involvement, 144t
Lyme disease, 144t, 151, 156t, 163, 192
Lymphoid hypertrophy, 95

Macrocephaly ("large head"), 100, 101, 126–27, 128t
Macrocrania, 126–27, 127t
Macro-orchidism, 95
Magnesium supplements, 193
Maple syrup urine disease, 108t, 128t
Megalencephaly
   autosomal dominant, 129t
   causes of, 128t–129t
   Krabbe disease and, 128t
   macrocephaly with, 127, 128t
   macrocrania without, 127t
Meningitis
   chronic, 191
   chronic daily headache and, 191, 193
   febrile seizures and, 41
   Lyme disease and, 192
Merosin-deficient muscular dystrophy, 90t
Metabolic myopathies, 77
Metachromic leukodystrophy, 129t
Methylmalonic acidurias, 108t
Mevalonic aciduria, 128t
Microangiopathic vasculitis, 144t
Midazolam
   for alternating hemiplegia, 11
   for status epilepticus, 63t
Migraine/migraine-like headache, 36, 135, 191–93

Miller Fisher syndrome, 162–63
Minicore disease, 77
Mixed axonal/demyelinative neuropathy, 72
Moyamoya disease, 135–37, 136f
Mucopolysaccharidoses, 129t
Multiple sclerosis/ADEM, 144t
Multiplex congenita, 76
Muscle-eye brain (Santavuori) syndrome, 90t
Muscular dystrophies of childhood, 90t
Myasthenia gravis, 121
Myoclonic encephalopathy of infants. *See* opsoclonus-myoclonus syndrome
Myoclonic seizures, 17, 18t, 48, 55, 135
Myotonic dystrophy type 1 (DM1), 79
Myotonic dystrophy type 2 (DM2), 79
Myotubular myopathy, 77

Nemaline rod myopathy, 77
Neonatal encephalopathy with seizures, 107
Neural tube defects, 130
Neuroblastoma, 162, 167–68
Neuroblastoma-associated opsoclonus-myoclonus syndrome, 168
Neurofibromatosis (NF), 100–103
   café-au-lait spots in, 100, 101f
   diagnostic criteria, 101
   macrocephaly in, 100, 101, 126
   megalencephaly and, 129t
   Moyamoya malformations and, 137
   type 1, 101–2, 129t
   type 2, 102
Neuromyelitis optica (device disease), 156t
Neuropathy rubric, 71t
NMDA receptor AB encephalopathy, 143–45, 144t
Nocturnal seizure, 23–24, 25
Non-dystrophin-related disorders, 90t
Nonspecific febrile illness, 64
Nystagmus, 10

Obsessive-compulsive disorder
    (OCD), 179–80
Obstructive hydrocephalus, 128t
Opsoclonus-myoclonus syndrome,
    162, 167–68
Optic glioma, 101, 102
Ornithine transcarbamylase (OTC)
    deficiency, 107–10, 108t, 109f
Oxcarbazepine, 24

Pallid infantile syncope, 29–31, 30t
Panayiotopoulos syndrome, 35–36
PANDAS (pediatric autoimmune disorders
    associated with streptococcal
    infection), 179
Paroxysmal kinesogenic
    choreoathetosis, 84t
Paroxysmal nonkinesigenic
    choreoathetosis, 84t
Paroxysmal torticollis of infancy, 84t
Pentobarbital, 63, 63t
Phenobarbital
    for ornithine transcarbamylase
        deficiency, 107
    for partial seizures, 24
    for status epilepticus, 62–63, 63t
Physical therapy
    for Charcot Marie Tooth disorders, 72
    for Duchenne muscular dystrophy, 91
    for myotonic dystrophy, 79
    for neurofibromatosis, 102
Plexiform neurofibroma, 101, 102
Post-staring impairment, 7t
Prednisone
    for Duchenne muscular dystrophy, 91
    for NMDA receptor AB
        encephalopathy, 143
    for opsoclonus-myoclonus syndrome, 167
Propionic aciduria, 108t
Psychogenic movement disorder, 185
"Purple glove" syndrome (venous
    sclerosis), 62
Pyridoxine dependency, 108t

Rett syndrome, 115–18
    diagnostic criteria, exclusion, 116t
    stages and treatment, 117
    treatment, 117
Rituximab
    for device disease, 156t
    for NMDA receptor autoimmune
        encephalitis, 144
    for opsoclonus-myoclonus
        syndrome, 168

Santavuori (muscle-eye brain)
    syndrome, 90t
Segawa disease (hereditary progressive
    dystonia with diurnal
    variation), 83, 85
Seizures
    absence, 4–7, 55, 56f, 57, 177–78
    autonomic, 35
    clonic, 17, 18t, 30t, 35, 55, 135
    clonic-tonic-clonic seizures, 55
    daytime, 24
    febrile, 41–42
    focal, 4–7, 41, 144
    myoclonic, 17, 18t, 48, 55, 135
    neonatal, as a function of age, 108t
    neonatal encephalopathy with, 107
    nocturnal, 23–24
    in Rett syndrome, 117
    tonic, 30t, 35, 48, 50, 135
    tonic-clonic, 24, 30t, 35, 39, 41, 55,
        57–58, 61, 93
Sensory deficits, 154, 186, 187
Serotonin-norepinephrine reuptake
    inhibitors (SNRIs), 193
Sickle cell disease, 137
Sinovenous thrombosis, 191
Sotos syndrome, 129t
Spina bifida, 173
Spinal muscular atrophy (SMA), 121–23
Staring, 4–5, 7t. See also absence seizures
Status epilepticus, 62–64
    drug treatment, 63t

Subarachnoid hemorrhage, 108*t*
Subdural hematoma, 162*t*, 186, 191
Sunsetting, with downward deviation of the eyes, 130

Tethered cord, 173–75
   MRI, 174*f*
Tics/Tourette syndrome, 179–80
Toe walking
   in Duchenne muscular dystrophy, 88
   in tethered cord, 173, 174*f*
Tonic-clonic seizures, 24, 30*t*, 35, 39, 41, 55, 57–58, 61, 93
Tonic seizures, 30*t*, 35, 48, 50, 135
Topiramate
   for chronic migraine headache, 192
   for partial seizures, 24
Transient motor tic disorder, 180
Transverse myelitis, 154–57
   differential diagnosis, with supportive MRI findings, 156*t*
Tricyclic antidepressants, 193
Tuberous sclerosis, 49, 129*t*

Unilateral left hemisphere hydrocephalus due to obstruction of the foramen of Monro, 130*f*
Urea cycle disorders, 110

VACTERL syndrome, 130
Valproate
   for absence seizures, 6
   for chronic migraine headache, 193
   for juvenile myoclonic epilepsy, 57
   for status epilepticus, 63t
Valproic acid
   for partial seizures, 24
   for status epilepticus, 63
Valproic acid-induced liver toxicity, 63
Venous sclerosis ("purple glove" syndrome), 62
Vigabatrin, 49
Viral encephalitides, 144*t*
Vitamin B2/riboflavin supplements, 193
Vitamin D supplements, 193

Walker-Warburg syndrome, 90*t*
Werdnig-Hoffman disease, 122
West's syndrome, 48

X-linked CMT disease, 70, 72

Made in the USA
Monee, IL
03 May 2026